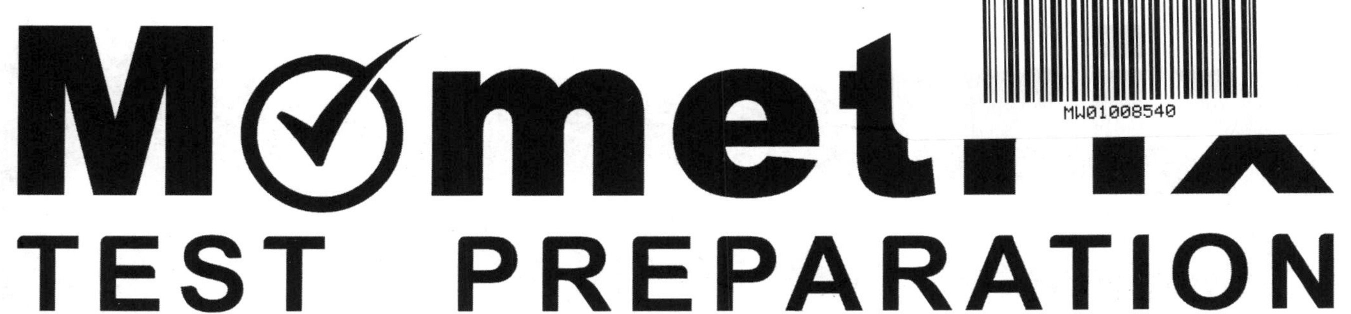

Certified Coding Specialist Exam Secrets Study Guide

DEAR FUTURE EXAM SUCCESS STORY

First of all, **THANK YOU** for purchasing Mometrix study materials!

Second, congratulations! You are one of the few determined test-takers who are committed to doing whatever it takes to excel on your exam. **You have come to the right place.** We developed these study materials with one goal in mind: to deliver you the information you need in a format that's concise and easy to use.

In addition to optimizing your guide for the content of the test, we've outlined our recommended steps for breaking down the preparation process into small, attainable goals so you can make sure you stay on track.

We've also analyzed the entire test-taking process, identifying the most common pitfalls and showing how you can overcome them and be ready for any curveball the test throws you.

Standardized testing is one of the biggest obstacles on your road to success, which only increases the importance of doing well in the high-pressure, high-stakes environment of test day. Your results on this test could have a significant impact on your future, and this guide provides the information and practical advice to help you achieve your full potential on test day.

Your success is our success

We would love to hear from you! If you would like to share the story of your exam success or if you have any questions or comments in regard to our products, please contact us at **800-673-8175** or **support@mometrix.com**.

Thanks again for your business and we wish you continued success!

Sincerely,
The Mometrix Test Preparation Team

Need more help? Check out our flashcards at:
http://MometrixFlashcards.com/CodingSpecialist

Written and edited by the Mometrix Exam Secrets Test Prep Team
Printed in the United States of America

TABLE OF CONTENTS

Introduction

Thank you for purchasing this resource! You have made the choice to prepare yourself for a test that could have a huge impact on your future, and this guide is designed to help you be fully ready for test day. Obviously, it's important to have a solid understanding of the test material, but you also need to be prepared for the unique environment and stressors of the test, so that you can perform to the best of your abilities.

For this purpose, the first section that appears in this guide is the **Secret Keys**. We've devoted countless hours to meticulously researching what works and what doesn't, and we've boiled down our findings to the five most impactful steps you can take to improve your performance on the test. We start at the beginning with study planning and move through the preparation process, all the way to the testing strategies that will help you get the most out of what you know when you're finally sitting in front of the test.

We recommend that you start preparing for your test as far in advance as possible. However, if you've bought this guide as a last-minute study resource and only have a few days before your test, we recommend that you skip over the first two Secret Keys since they address a long-term study plan.

If you struggle with **test anxiety**, we strongly encourage you to check out our recommendations for how you can overcome it. Test anxiety is a formidable foe, but it can be beaten, and we want to make sure you have the tools you need to defeat it.

Secret Key #1 – Plan Big, Study Small

There's a lot riding on your performance. If you want to ace this test, you're going to need to keep your skills sharp and the material fresh in your mind. You need a plan that lets you review everything you need to know while still fitting in your schedule. We'll break this strategy down into three categories.

Information Organization

Start with the information you already have: the official test outline. From this, you can make a complete list of all the concepts you need to cover before the test. Organize these concepts into groups that can be studied together, and create a list of any related vocabulary you need to learn so you can brush up on any difficult terms. You'll want to keep this vocabulary list handy once you actually start studying since you may need to add to it along the way.

Time Management

Once you have your set of study concepts, decide how to spread them out over the time you have left before the test. Break your study plan into small, clear goals so you have a manageable task for each day and know exactly what you're doing. Then just focus on one small step at a time. When you manage your time this way, you don't need to spend hours at a time studying. Studying a small block of content for a short period each day helps you retain information better and avoid stressing over how much you have left to do. You can relax knowing that you have a plan to cover everything in time. In order for this strategy to be effective though, you have to start studying early and stick to your schedule. Avoid the exhaustion and futility that comes from last-minute cramming!

Study Environment

The environment you study in has a big impact on your learning. Studying in a coffee shop, while probably more enjoyable, is not likely to be as fruitful as studying in a quiet room. It's important to keep distractions to a minimum. You're only planning to study for a short block of time, so make the most of it. Don't pause to check your phone or get up to find a snack. It's also important to **avoid multitasking**. Research has consistently shown that multitasking will make your studying dramatically less effective. Your study area should also be comfortable and well-lit so you don't have the distraction of straining your eyes or sitting on an uncomfortable chair.

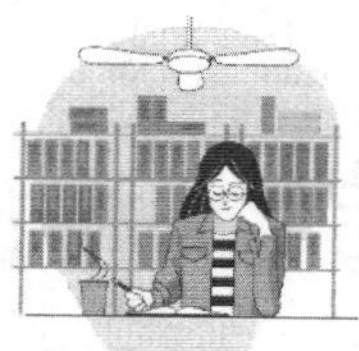

The time of day you study is also important. You want to be rested and alert. Don't wait until just before bedtime. Study when you'll be most likely to comprehend and remember. Even better, if you know what time of day your test will be, set that time aside for study. That way your brain will be used to working on that subject at that specific time and you'll have a better chance of recalling information.

Finally, it can be helpful to team up with others who are studying for the same test. Your actual studying should be done in as isolated an environment as possible, but the work of organizing the information and setting up the study plan can be divided up. In between study sessions, you can discuss with your teammates the concepts that you're all studying and quiz each other on the details. Just be sure that your teammates are as serious about the test as you are. If you find that your study time is being replaced with social time, you might need to find a new team.

Secret Key #2 – Make Your Studying Count

You're devoting a lot of time and effort to preparing for this test, so you want to be absolutely certain it will pay off. This means doing more than just reading the content and hoping you can remember it on test day. It's important to make every minute of study count. There are two main areas you can focus on to make your studying count.

Retention

It doesn't matter how much time you study if you can't remember the material. You need to make sure you are retaining the concepts. To check your retention of the information you're learning, try recalling it at later times with minimal prompting. Try carrying around flashcards and glance at one or two from time to time or ask a friend who's also studying for the test to quiz you.

To enhance your retention, look for ways to put the information into practice so that you can apply it rather than simply recalling it. If you're using the information in practical ways, it will be much easier to remember. Similarly, it helps to solidify a concept in your mind if you're not only reading it to yourself but also explaining it to someone else. Ask a friend to let you teach them about a concept you're a little shaky on (or speak aloud to an imaginary audience if necessary). As you try to summarize, define, give examples, and answer your friend's questions, you'll understand the concepts better and they will stay with you longer. Finally, step back for a big picture view and ask yourself how each piece of information fits with the whole subject. When you link the different concepts together and see them working together as a whole, it's easier to remember the individual components.

Finally, practice showing your work on any multi-step problems, even if you're just studying. Writing out each step you take to solve a problem will help solidify the process in your mind, and you'll be more likely to remember it during the test.

Modality

Modality simply refers to the means or method by which you study. Choosing a study modality that fits your own individual learning style is crucial. No two people learn best in exactly the same way, so it's important to know your strengths and use them to your advantage.

For example, if you learn best by visualization, focus on visualizing a concept in your mind and draw an image or a diagram. Try color-coding your notes, illustrating them, or creating symbols that will trigger your mind to recall a learned concept. If you learn best by hearing or discussing information, find a study partner who learns the same way or read aloud to yourself. Think about how to put the information in your own words. Imagine that you are giving a lecture on the topic and record yourself so you can listen to it later.

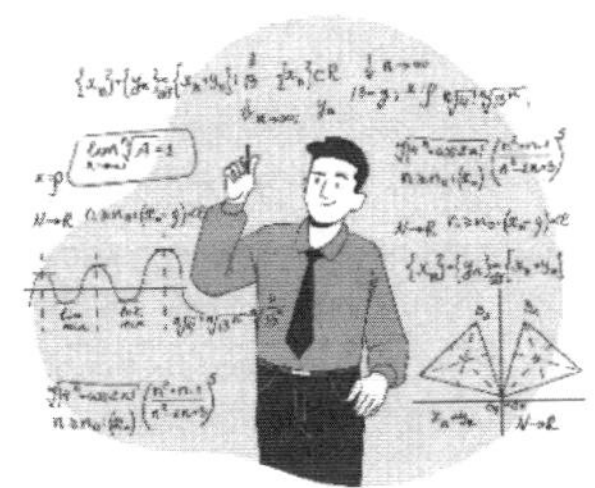

For any learning style, flashcards can be helpful. Organize the information so you can take advantage of spare moments to review. Underline key words or phrases. Use different colors for different categories. Mnemonic devices (such as creating a short list in which every item starts with the same letter) can also help with retention. Find what works best for you and use it to store the information in your mind most effectively and easily.

Secret Key #3 – Practice the Right Way

Your success on test day depends not only on how many hours you put into preparing, but also on whether you prepared the right way. It's good to check along the way to see if your studying is paying off. One of the most effective ways to do this is by taking practice tests to evaluate your progress. Practice tests are useful because they show exactly where you need to improve. Every time you take a practice test, pay special attention to these three groups of questions:

- The questions you got wrong
- The questions you had to guess on, even if you guessed right
- The questions you found difficult or slow to work through

This will show you exactly what your weak areas are, and where you need to devote more study time. Ask yourself why each of these questions gave you trouble. Was it because you didn't understand the material? Was it because you didn't remember the vocabulary? Do you need more repetitions on this type of question to build speed and confidence? Dig into those questions and figure out how you can strengthen your weak areas as you go back to review the material.

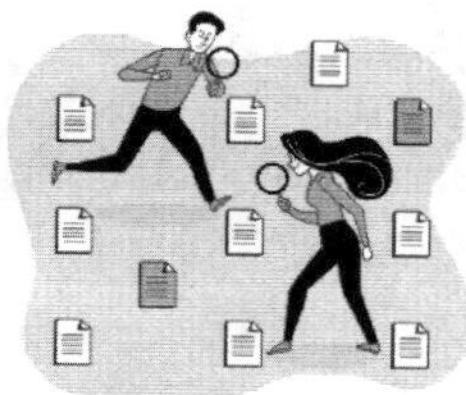

Additionally, many practice tests have a section explaining the answer choices. It can be tempting to read the explanation and think that you now have a good understanding of the concept. However, an explanation likely only covers part of the question's broader context. Even if the explanation makes perfect sense, **go back and investigate** every concept related to the question until you're positive you have a thorough understanding.

As you go along, keep in mind that the practice test is just that: practice. Memorizing these questions and answers will not be very helpful on the actual test because it is unlikely to have any of the same exact questions. If you only know the right answers to the sample questions, you won't be prepared for the real thing. **Study the concepts** until you understand them fully, and then you'll be able to answer any question that shows up on the test.

It's important to wait on the practice tests until you're ready. If you take a test on your first day of study, you may be overwhelmed by the amount of material covered and how much you need to learn. Work up to it gradually.

On test day, you'll need to be prepared for answering questions, managing your time, and using the test-taking strategies you've learned. It's a lot to balance, like a mental marathon that will have a big impact on your future. Like training for a marathon, you'll need to start slowly and work your way up. When test day arrives, you'll be ready.

Start with the strategies you've read in the first two Secret Keys—plan your course and study in the way that works best for you. If you have time, consider using multiple study resources to get different approaches to the same concepts. It can be helpful to see difficult concepts from more than one angle. Then find a good source for practice tests. Many times, the test website will suggest potential study resources or provide sample tests.

Practice Test Strategy

If you're able to find at least three practice tests, we recommend this strategy:

Untimed and Open-Book Practice

Take the first test with no time constraints and with your notes and study guide handy. Take your time and focus on applying the strategies you've learned.

Timed and Open-Book Practice

Take the second practice test open-book as well, but set a timer and practice pacing yourself to finish in time.

Timed and Closed-Book Practice

Take any other practice tests as if it were test day. Set a timer and put away your study materials. Sit at a table or desk in a quiet room, imagine yourself at the testing center, and answer questions as quickly and accurately as possible.

Keep repeating timed and closed-book tests on a regular basis until you run out of practice tests or it's time for the actual test. Your mind will be ready for the schedule and stress of test day, and you'll be able to focus on recalling the material you've learned.

Secret Key #4 – Pace Yourself

Once you're fully prepared for the material on the test, your biggest challenge on test day will be managing your time. Just knowing that the clock is ticking can make you panic even if you have plenty of time left. Work on pacing yourself so you can build confidence against the time constraints of the exam. Pacing is a difficult skill to master, especially in a high-pressure environment, so **practice is vital**.

Set time expectations for your pace based on how much time is available. For example, if a section has 60 questions and the time limit is 30 minutes, you know you have to average 30 seconds or less per question in order to answer them all. Although 30 seconds is the hard limit, set 25 seconds per question as your goal, so you reserve extra time to spend on harder questions. When you budget extra time for the harder questions, you no longer have any reason to stress when those questions take longer to answer.

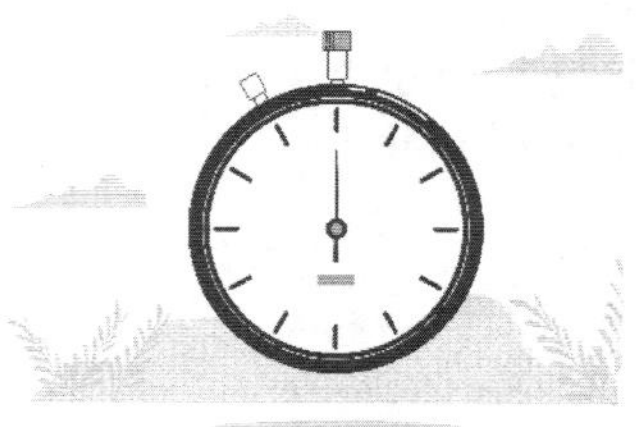

Don't let this time expectation distract you from working through the test at a calm, steady pace, but keep it in mind so you don't spend too much time on any one question. Recognize that taking extra time on one question you don't understand may keep you from answering two that you do understand later in the test. If your time limit for a question is up and you're still not sure of the answer, mark it and move on, and come back to it later if the time and the test format allow. If the testing format doesn't allow you to return to earlier questions, just make an educated guess; then put it out of your mind and move on.

On the easier questions, be careful not to rush. It may seem wise to hurry through them so you have more time for the challenging ones, but it's not worth missing one if you know the concept and just didn't take the time to read the question fully. Work efficiently but make sure you understand the question and have looked at all of the answer choices, since more than one may seem right at first.

Even if you're paying attention to the time, you may find yourself a little behind at some point. You should speed up to get back on track, but do so wisely. Don't panic; just take a few seconds less on each question until you're caught up. Don't guess without thinking, but do look through the answer choices and eliminate any you know are wrong. If you can get down to two choices, it is often worthwhile to guess from those. Once you've chosen an answer, move on and don't dwell on any that you skipped or had to hurry through. If a question was taking too long, chances are it was one of the harder ones, so you weren't as likely to get it right anyway.

On the other hand, if you find yourself getting ahead of schedule, it may be beneficial to slow down a little. The more quickly you work, the more likely you are to make a careless mistake that will affect your score. You've budgeted time for each question, so don't be afraid to spend that time. Practice an efficient but careful pace to get the most out of the time you have.

Secret Key #5 – Have a Plan for Guessing

When you're taking the test, you may find yourself stuck on a question. Some of the answer choices seem better than others, but you don't see the one answer choice that is obviously correct. What do you do?

The scenario described above is very common, yet most test takers have not effectively prepared for it. Developing and practicing a plan for guessing may be one of the single most effective uses of your time as you get ready for the exam.

In developing your plan for guessing, there are three questions to address:

- When should you start the guessing process?
- How should you narrow down the choices?
- Which answer should you choose?

When to Start the Guessing Process

Unless your plan for guessing is to select C every time (which, despite its merits, is not what we recommend), you need to leave yourself enough time to apply your answer elimination strategies. Since you have a limited amount of time for each question, that means that if you're going to give yourself the best shot at guessing correctly, you have to decide quickly whether or not you will guess.

Of course, the best-case scenario is that you don't have to guess at all, so first, see if you can answer the question based on your knowledge of the subject and basic reasoning skills. Focus on the key words in the question and try to jog your memory of related topics. Give yourself a chance to bring the knowledge to mind, but once you realize that you don't have (or you can't access) the knowledge you need to answer the question, it's time to start the guessing process.

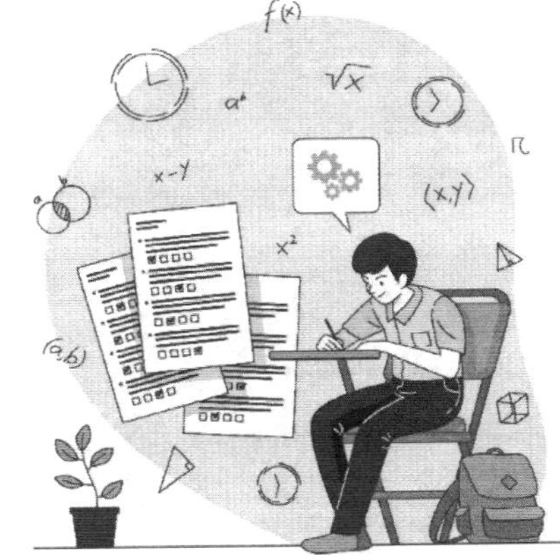

It's almost always better to start the guessing process too early than too late. It only takes a few seconds to remember something and answer the question from knowledge. Carefully eliminating wrong answer choices takes longer. Plus, going through the process of eliminating answer choices can actually help jog your memory.

Summary: Start the guessing process as soon as you decide that you can't answer the question based on your knowledge.

How to Narrow Down the Choices

The next chapter in this book (**Test-Taking Strategies**) includes a wide range of strategies for how to approach questions and how to look for answer choices to eliminate. You will definitely want to read those carefully, practice them, and figure out which ones work best for you. Here though, we're going to address a mindset rather than a particular strategy.

Your odds of guessing an answer correctly depend on how many options you are choosing from.

Number of options left	5	4	3	2	1
Odds of guessing correctly	20%	25%	33%	50%	100%

You can see from this chart just how valuable it is to be able to eliminate incorrect answers and make an educated guess, but there are two things that many test takers do that cause them to miss out on the benefits of guessing:

- Accidentally eliminating the correct answer
- Selecting an answer based on an impression

We'll look at the first one here, and the second one in the next section.

To avoid accidentally eliminating the correct answer, we recommend a thought exercise called **the $5 challenge**. In this challenge, you only eliminate an answer choice from contention if you are willing to bet $5 on it being wrong. Why $5? Five dollars is a small but not insignificant amount of money. It's an amount you could afford to lose but wouldn't want to throw away. And while losing $5 once might not hurt too much, doing it twenty times will set you back $100. In the same way, each small decision you make—eliminating a choice here, guessing on a question there—won't by itself impact your score very much, but when you put them all together, they can make a big difference. By holding each answer choice elimination decision to a higher standard, you can reduce the risk of accidentally eliminating the correct answer.

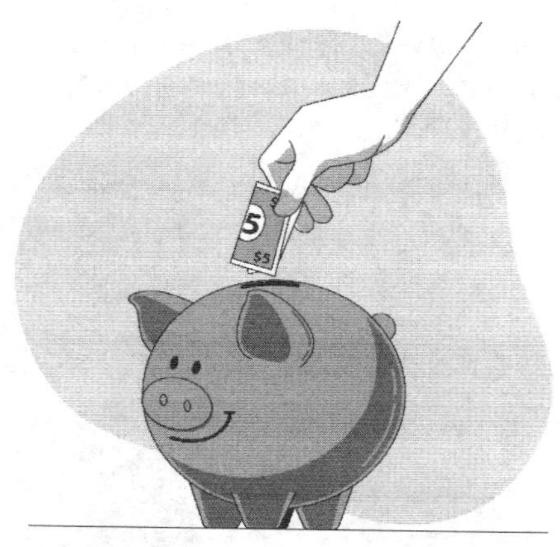

The $5 challenge can also be applied in a positive sense: If you are willing to bet $5 that an answer choice *is* correct, go ahead and mark it as correct.

Summary: Only eliminate an answer choice if you are willing to bet $5 that it is wrong.

Which Answer to Choose

You're taking the test. You've run into a hard question and decided you'll have to guess. You've eliminated all the answer choices you're willing to bet $5 on. Now you have to pick an answer. Why do we even need to talk about this? Why can't you just pick whichever one you feel like when the time comes?

The answer to these questions is that if you don't come into the test with a plan, you'll rely on your impression to select an answer choice, and if you do that, you risk falling into a trap. The test writers know that everyone who takes their test will be guessing on some of the questions, so they intentionally write wrong answer choices to seem plausible. You still have to pick an answer though, and if the wrong answer choices are designed to look right, how can you ever be sure that you're not falling for their trap? The best solution we've found to this dilemma is to take the decision out of your hands entirely. Here is the process we recommend:

Once you've eliminated any choices that you are confident (willing to bet $5) are wrong, select the first remaining choice as your answer.

Whether you choose to select the first remaining choice, the second, or the last, the important thing is that you use some preselected standard. Using this approach guarantees that you will not be enticed into selecting an answer choice that looks right, because you are not basing your decision on how the answer choices look.

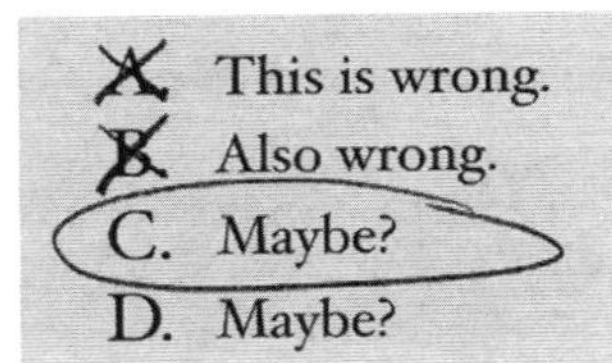

This is not meant to make you question your knowledge. Instead, it is to help you recognize the difference between your knowledge and your impressions. There's a huge difference between thinking an answer is right because of what you know, and thinking an answer is right because it looks or sounds like it should be right.

Summary: To ensure that your selection is appropriately random, make a predetermined selection from among all answer choices you have not eliminated.

Test-Taking Strategies

This section contains a list of test-taking strategies that you may find helpful as you work through the test. By taking what you know and applying logical thought, you can maximize your chances of answering any question correctly!

It is very important to realize that every question is different and every person is different: no single strategy will work on every question, and no single strategy will work for every person. That's why we've included all of them here, so you can try them out and determine which ones work best for different types of questions and which ones work best for you.

Question Strategies

✓ Read Carefully

Read the question and the answer choices carefully. Don't miss the question because you misread the terms. You have plenty of time to read each question thoroughly and make sure you understand what is being asked. Yet a happy medium must be attained, so don't waste too much time. You must read carefully and efficiently.

✓ Contextual Clues

Look for contextual clues. If the question includes a word you are not familiar with, look at the immediate context for some indication of what the word might mean. Contextual clues can often give you all the information you need to decipher the meaning of an unfamiliar word. Even if you can't determine the meaning, you may be able to narrow down the possibilities enough to make a solid guess at the answer to the question.

✓ Prefixes

If you're having trouble with a word in the question or answer choices, try dissecting it. Take advantage of every clue that the word might include. Prefixes and suffixes can be a huge help. Usually, they allow you to determine a basic meaning. *Pre-* means before, *post-* means after, *pro-* is positive, *de-* is negative. From prefixes and suffixes, you can get an idea of the general meaning of the word and try to put it into context.

✓ Hedge Words

Watch out for critical hedge words, such as *likely, may, can, sometimes, often, almost, mostly, usually, generally, rarely,* and *sometimes.* Question writers insert these hedge phrases to cover every possibility. Often an answer choice will be wrong simply because it leaves no room for exception. Be on guard for answer choices that have definitive words such as *exactly* and *always.*

✓ Switchback Words

Stay alert for *switchbacks.* These are the words and phrases frequently used to alert you to shifts in thought. The most common switchback words are *but, although,* and *however.* Others include *nevertheless, on the other hand, even though, while, in spite of, despite,* and *regardless of.* Switchback words are important to catch because they can change the direction of the question or an answer choice.

✓ Face Value

When in doubt, use common sense. Accept the situation in the problem at face value. Don't read too much into it. These problems will not require you to make wild assumptions. If you have to go beyond creativity and warp time or space in order to have an answer choice fit the question, then you should move on and consider the other answer choices. These are normal problems rooted in reality. The applicable relationship or explanation may not be readily apparent, but it is there for you to figure out. Use your common sense to interpret anything that isn't clear.

Answer Choice Strategies

✓ Answer Selection

The most thorough way to pick an answer choice is to identify and eliminate wrong answers until only one is left, then confirm it is the correct answer. Sometimes an answer choice may immediately seem right, but be careful. The test writers will usually put more than one reasonable answer choice on each question, so take a second to read all of them and make sure that the other choices are not equally obvious. As long as you have time left, it is better to read every answer choice than to pick the first one that looks right without checking the others.

✓ Answer Choice Families

An answer choice family consists of two (in rare cases, three) answer choices that are very similar in construction and cannot all be true at the same time. If you see two answer choices that are direct opposites or parallels, one of them is usually the correct answer. For instance, if one answer choice says that quantity *x* increases and another either says that quantity *x* decreases (opposite) or says that quantity *y* increases (parallel), then those answer choices would fall into the same family. An answer choice that doesn't match the construction of the answer choice family is more likely to be incorrect. Most questions will not have answer choice families, but when they do appear, you should be prepared to recognize them.

✓ Eliminate Answers

Eliminate answer choices as soon as you realize they are wrong, but make sure you consider all possibilities. If you are eliminating answer choices and realize that the last one you are left with is also wrong, don't panic. Start over and consider each choice again. There may be something you missed the first time that you will realize on the second pass.

✓ Avoid Fact Traps

Don't be distracted by an answer choice that is factually true but doesn't answer the question. You are looking for the choice that answers the question. Stay focused on what the question is asking for so you don't accidentally pick an answer that is true but incorrect. Always go back to the question and make sure the answer choice you've selected actually answers the question and is not merely a true statement.

✓ Extreme Statements

In general, you should avoid answers that put forth extreme actions as standard practice or proclaim controversial ideas as established fact. An answer choice that states the "process should be used in certain situations, if…" is much more likely to be correct than one that states the "process should be discontinued completely." The first is a calm rational statement and doesn't even make a definitive, uncompromising stance, using a hedge word *if* to provide wiggle room, whereas the second choice is far more extreme.

✓ Benchmark

As you read through the answer choices and you come across one that seems to answer the question well, mentally select that answer choice. This is not your final answer, but it's the one that will help you evaluate the other answer choices. The one that you selected is your benchmark or standard for judging each of the other answer choices. Every other answer choice must be compared to your benchmark. That choice is correct until proven otherwise by another answer choice beating it. If you find a better answer, then that one becomes your new benchmark. Once you've decided that no other choice answers the question as well as your benchmark, you have your final answer.

✓ Predict the Answer

Before you even start looking at the answer choices, it is often best to try to predict the answer. When you come up with the answer on your own, it is easier to avoid distractions and traps because you will know exactly what to look for. The right answer choice is unlikely to be word-for-word what you came up with, but it should be a close match. Even if you are confident that you have the right answer, you should still take the time to read each option before moving on.

General Strategies

✓ Tough Questions

If you are stumped on a problem or it appears too hard or too difficult, don't waste time. Move on! Remember though, if you can quickly check for obviously incorrect answer choices, your chances of guessing correctly are greatly improved. Before you completely give up, at least try to knock out a couple of possible answers. Eliminate what you can and then guess at the remaining answer choices before moving on.

✓ Check Your Work

Since you will probably not know every term listed and the answer to every question, it is important that you get credit for the ones that you do know. Don't miss any questions through careless mistakes. If at all possible, try to take a second to look back over your answer selection and make sure you've selected the correct answer choice and haven't made a costly careless mistake (such as marking an answer choice that you didn't mean to mark). This quick double check should more than pay for itself in caught mistakes for the time it costs.

✓ Pace Yourself

It's easy to be overwhelmed when you're looking at a page full of questions; your mind is confused and full of random thoughts, and the clock is ticking down faster than you would like. Calm down and maintain the pace that you have set for yourself. Especially as you get down to the last few minutes of the test, don't let the small numbers on the clock make you panic. As long as you are on track by monitoring your pace, you are guaranteed to have time for each question.

✓ Don't Rush

It is very easy to make errors when you are in a hurry. Maintaining a fast pace in answering questions is pointless if it makes you miss questions that you would have gotten right otherwise. Test writers like to include distracting information and wrong answers that seem right. Taking a little extra time to avoid careless mistakes can make all the difference in your test score. Find a pace that allows you to be confident in the answers that you select.

⊘ KEEP MOVING

Panicking will not help you pass the test, so do your best to stay calm and keep moving. Taking deep breaths and going through the answer elimination steps you practiced can help to break through a stress barrier and keep your pace.

Final Notes

The combination of a solid foundation of content knowledge and the confidence that comes from practicing your plan for applying that knowledge is the key to maximizing your performance on test day. As your foundation of content knowledge is built up and strengthened, you'll find that the strategies included in this chapter become more and more effective in helping you quickly sift through the distractions and traps of the test to isolate the correct answer.

Now that you're preparing to move forward into the test content chapters of this book, be sure to keep your goal in mind. As you read, think about how you will be able to apply this information on the test. If you've already seen sample questions for the test and you have an idea of the question format and style, try to come up with questions of your own that you can answer based on what you're reading. This will give you valuable practice applying your knowledge in the same ways you can expect to on test day.

Good luck and good studying!

Coding Knowledge and Skills

Documentation in the Health Record

Reporting Symptoms

A symptom is reported when a definitive diagnosis is not made by the provider. For example, if the documentation only states that the patient presents with a cough and fever, the codes for cough and fever should be reported. However, when a definitive diagnosis is made by the provider and the documented signs and/or symptoms are inclusive to that diagnosis, do not report the signs and/or symptoms. For example, if the documentation states that the patient has the flu, a cough, and a fever, only the code representing the flu would be reported because the cough and fever are inclusive symptoms of the definitive flu diagnosis. The symptom codes can be found in Chapter 18 of the *International Classification of Diseases, Tenth Revision, Clinical Modification* (ICD-10-CM), "Symptoms, Signs, and Abnormal Clinical and Laboratory Findings, Not Elsewhere Classified."

Initial and Subsequent Treatment of Injury and Treatment of Sequela of Injury

Initial treatment is active care directed at the injury with the purpose of healing it, and it often involves the development of a plan of care. Take, for example, a broken ankle. The initial treatment might involve immobilization, a visit to the ED, or an X-ray to evaluate the extent of the break. Subsequent treatment indicates that the care is routine. At this stage, the injury is viewed as being in the recovery phase. Subsequent treatment could be physical therapy to strengthen the muscles surrounding the ankle. A sequela is a complication and/or condition that stems from the original injury. A sequela of a broken ankle might be chronic pain, for which a provider might deem it necessary to prescribe opioids on a long-term basis.

Screening, Diagnostic, and Therapeutic Procedures

A **screening procedure** is considered routine based on a patient's risk factors, such as age and family history. A common routine screening procedure may be a colonoscopy for a patient with a family history of colorectal cancer. A **diagnostic procedure** is done with the intent to rule out or determine a diagnosis based on the images or findings obtained from the procedure. Usually, the patient will exhibit signs or symptoms that deem the procedure as being medically necessary. An example of a diagnostic procedure may be a colonoscopy to determine the root cause of rectal bleeding. A **therapeutic procedure** is one that is aimed at treating an already-established disease or condition, such as removing a polyp or lesion.

Presumptive and Definitive Drug Tests

A **presumptive drug test** reports if the body system is positive or negative for a general drug class. For example, a presumptive drug test may be ordered to determine the presence of opioids. A **definitive drug test** will analyze the specific agent and/or how much of that agent is in the body. If a presumptive drug test is positive for opioids, a definitive test will elaborate on the type of opiate it is, such as codeine or oxycodone, and the specific amount within the body. Presumptive drug testing services may be reported with CPT codes 80305–80307, and definitive drug testing services may be reported with Current Procedural Terminology (CPT) codes 80320–80377 or with Healthcare Common Procedure Coding System (HCPCS) codes G0480–G0483 and G0659.

Billing of Separate Evaluation and Management During Postoperative Global Period

The postoperative global period is defined by Medicare as "the necessary services normally furnished by a surgeon before, during, and after a procedure." This would include services such as biopsy results, follow-up incision care, and any postoperative complications arising from the initial procedure. If an unrelated condition arises during the postoperative global period that requires care, that service can be separately reportable. For example, the findings from a diagnostic procedure show an illness that requires immediate medical attention. Any treatment directed to that condition would be considered unrelated to postoperative care and would be billable.

Identifying Causal Relationship Between Diagnoses

The term "with" that is sometimes located in the description of a diagnosis implies that a **causal** relationship exists between two or more conditions, even if the provider's documentation does not specifically link them as being related. On the other hand, if the provider specifically documents that the two conditions are unrelated, they would be reported in that manner. The most common presumed diagnosis relationships would be hypertension with chronic heart disease and hypertension with kidney disease, along with diabetes and the many complications that stem from it.

Billing Separate E/M Codes with Procedures

If the history intake and examination are **unrelated** to the procedure being performed, a separate E/M code may be reported separately because it is significantly identifiable. For example, a patient has a biopsy after presenting with an abnormal lesion. During that same encounter, the patient also complains of flu-like symptoms and a nasal swab is collected to determine if the flu virus is present. Because the flu-like symptoms are unrelated to the biopsy of an abnormal lesion, an E/M code may be reported. In this case, a modifier should be used to indicate that two services were provided to the patient by the same physician on the same day.

ICD-10-CM Manual Features for Ensuring Proper Coding Techniques

Contained in the ICD-10-CM manual are many unique features to assist coding professionals in ensuring proper coding techniques. One of these features includes a "What's New" section, which highlights the different ICD-10-CM codes that have been added, removed, and revised for that fiscal year. "Conventions for the ICD-10-CM" in Section I can be reviewed to understand the definitions of all index notations, such as "With," "See Also," "Excludes1," and many others. This section also contains general coding guidelines that explain how to sequence acute and chronic conditions and the correct use of Z codes. The tables for neoplasms, external causes, and drugs and chemicals provide a visual guide aimed at assisting coders in their selection of these diagnoses. Additionally, chapter-specific guidelines with examples are provided at the beginning of each chapter throughout the manual to elaborate on and clarify sequencing and code selection related to that body system and/or injury.

CPT Manual Features for Ensuring Proper Coding Techniques

The CPT manual contains multiple appendices aimed at helping coding professionals select the most accurate procedure and/or E/M codes. For example, Appendix B lists all of the new, revised, and deleted CPT codes for the current fiscal year. If procedures were deleted or revised, Appendices D and F will provide a cross reference to where a similar, active procedure code is available. Appendix C is a useful tool that provides extended guidelines for the use of E/M services, which include the federal documentation guidelines set forth by the Centers for Medicare & Medicaid Services (CMS). Additionally, Appendices N, O, and P contain illustrations specific to nerves, vascular families, and interventional radiology. For a complete list of appendices, see the "Introduction" section of the CPT manual.

HCPCS Level II

HCPCS Level II was developed by CMS to represent medical supplies, medication, and physician and nonphysician services that are not covered within the CPT manual. If locating a code in the HCPCS Level II manual, begin by identifying the supply, medication, or service that the patient received and look up the term in the index. For example, outpatient services structured to promote sobriety would be considered rehabilitation. Locate "Rehabilitation" in the index. Under "Rehabilitation" is a list of related terms, such as "Pulmonary" and "Service." Select "Service." This subheading lists "Substance abuse," which is represented by HCPCS codes H2034–H2036. Be aware that the index alone is not a reliable guide to accurate coding. All codes and their guidelines should be reviewed in the appropriate section prior to their selection.

Locating Diagnosis Codes

If you are locating a diagnosis code in the ICD-10-CM manual, begin with the "Index to Diseases and Injuries" section, located in the back of the book, and search for the **root** of the illness, injury, or disease. For example, if identifying the code for a transverse colon polyp, first locate "Polyp" in the index. Under "Polyp" is a list of anatomical locations. Search for "Colon." This subheading lists the types of polyps, presents the associated symptoms, and gives the anatomical location of where within the colon the polyp can be located. Be aware that the index alone is not a reliable guide to accurate diagnosis coding. In this example, the index would lead the coder to D12.3, "Benign neoplasm of transverse colon." However, if the documentation does not specifically state that a polyp was adenomatous and/or benign, the notes below the code suggest that the choice selection should be unspecified, as represented by K63.5, "Polyp of colon."

Locating Procedure Codes

If you are locating a procedure code in the CPT manual, turn to the CPT Index section located in the back of the book. The index is organized by the **main term(s)** of a procedure. For example, if an open ankle arthrodesis were performed, "Arthrodesis" would be the main term to look for in the index. Under "Arthrodesis" is a list of anatomical locations. The entry for "Ankle" directs the coder to CPT code 27870. In this example, the description of CPT code 27870, "Arthrodesis, ankle, open," is the appropriate code selection. However, be aware that the index alone is not a reliable guide to accurate procedural coding. An additional code for arthrodesis of the proximal or distal tibiofibular joint is also listed but can only be found by turning to the correct CPT code section.

Primary Diagnosis and Procedure

Determining Primary Diagnosis Code When Multiple Conditions Are Documented

When multiple conditions exist, the primary diagnosis code will be **the foremost reason** that the patient is receiving treatment in a hospital setting. When two or more conditions are equally responsible for the admission, either may be chosen as the first listed code. Any coexisting chronic conditions that affect the current treatment may also be reported after the primary diagnosis. Chapter-specific guidelines do provide some insight into the exceptions to this rule. For example, if the reason for admission is an illness related to acquired immunodeficiency syndrome (AIDS), human immunodeficiency virus (HIV), or a malignancy and the patient also has one or more of these conditions, AIDS, HIV, and/or the malignancy will usually be listed first, even if the reason for the admission is a related illness.

Common Errors When Selecting Principal Diagnosis Code

In order to determine the principal diagnosis of a patient, the medical record needs to be reviewed in its entirety. Problems may arise in a hospital setting if a physician delays documenting a discharge summary because the coder must be able to understand which condition was ultimately responsible for an inpatient admission. If a provider's documentation is incomplete, unclear, or contradictory in any way, a coder must submit a query prior to selecting a diagnosis to ensure accuracy. When a provider is unresponsive, accurate code selection becomes challenging, if not impossible.

Coding When Time Spent on a Procedure Falls above or below the Description

Time spent toward a procedure can be counted when the midpoint has been passed. For example, if 15 minutes is the required time to bill a procedure, then at least 8 minutes must be documented by the provider. When the time spent falls in between two codes that are ranked in sequential typical times, report the code closest to the actual time. For example, if the provider documents 52 minutes, but the only codes available describe 45 minutes and 60 minutes, code to the 60 minutes because it is closest to the documented time.

Principal Procedure Code Selection When Multiple Procedures Are Documented

When multiple procedures are documented for a single encounter, a coding professional must review not only the type of procedures performed, but also the diagnoses associated with them. In general, a principal procedure is one that involves definitive treatment of the primary diagnosis of a patient. Any other diagnostic procedures would be reported as secondary with the applicable modifiers. On the other hand, if definitive treatment is given for a secondary diagnosis, and only diagnostic procedures were performed on the primary diagnosis, the diagnostic procedure would be considered principal because any procedures related to the primary diagnosis take priority.

Selecting Appropriate Diagnoses and Sequencing

Example Scenario

The initial encounter of a patient experiencing drug-induced tremors, which are caused by cyclosporine that the patient takes for anemia.

Because the primary reason for the visit is the drug-induced tremors, this will be the first-listed diagnosis code. Locate the root illness "Tremors" in the index of the ICD-10-CM manual. In the listing under this disease are the causes of tremors, which include G25.1, "Drug induced." Look up code G25.1 to verify accurate selection. In this particular section, the coder is directed to add a code to identify the drug causing the adverse reaction. Following the same process for "Adverse effect" will lead to the "Table of Drugs and Chemicals," in which the code for cyclosporine is T45.1X5A. The seventh character, A, is chosen to indicate active treatment. Next, search for "Anemia." Because no underlying condition is documented to be the cause for the anemia, select D64.9, "Anemia, unspecified." The correct coding for this encounter is then G25.1, T45.1X5A, D63.9.

Coding Conventions and Regulatory Guidance

Determining If Patient Is New or Established

A new patient is one who has not received treatment in the past 3 years from a physician or a different physician belonging to the same group practice of the exact same specialty or subspecialty. On the other hand, if a patient has received treatment in the past 3 years, from a physician or another physician belonging to the same group practice of the exact same specialty or subspecialty, he or she is considered to be an established patient. Even if the practice or provider moves to a different location, such as another state or to a different entity altogether, the patient would still be considered established if they have been treated by that physician within the past 3 years. For example, CPT codes 99201–99205 (evaluation of a new patient) may be reported for a patient seen in an endocrinology office for the first time. However, their follow-up with a different endocrinologist of the same practice 2 years later should be reported using CPT codes 99211–99215 (evaluation of an established patient).

Guidelines for Selecting Accurate E/M Service Codes

Medicare has established two sets of guidelines to assist coding professionals in selecting an accurate E/M service code. These are the 1995 and the 1997 E/M guidelines. The three components contained in these guidelines — history of present illness (HPI), examination, and medical decision making (MDM) — aid in determining which part of the medical record holds the most weight in medical necessity. When choosing the level of service, the guidelines cannot be combined. Rather, a coding professional should select the most advantageous guideline based on the medical documentation that they are reviewing.

1995 vs. 1997 E/M Guidelines

The first difference with these two sets of guidelines is the examination component. This component in the 1995 E/M guideline is considered generic and does not specify how to distinguish between an expanded problem-focused (limited) examination and a detailed (extended) examination for an affected body area or organ system. However, when the 1997 E/M guideline was released, the examination was very organ specific and included boxes and bullets of what was addressed during the examination. A second difference in these two guidelines is the HPI. The 1995 E/M guideline outlines that for an E/M to be considered extended or comprehensive partly based on the HPI, four or more elements addressing the chief complaint must be documented. However, in the 1997 E/M guideline, this may be overlooked if at least three chronic or inactive conditions are being addressed. Other portions of the guidelines, including the review of systems (ROS); past, family, and social history; and MDM remain the same between the two sets.

Elements of the HPI

The 1995 and 1997 E/M guidelines contain eight elements in the HPI portion. Below is a description of each element.

Element	Description	Examples
Location	Part of the body affected	Neck pain, nasal congestion
Severity	How serious the problem is	4/10 pain, deep laceration
Timing	When the problem occurs	Every 2 days, constantly
Modifying Factor	Steps taken to relieve the problem	Medication, ice/heat
Quality	Qualitative description of the problem	Sharp, clumpy
Duration	Onset of the problem	One week ago, last year
Context	Cause of the problem	Fall, car accident
Associated Signs/Symptoms	Related symptoms	Fever, dizziness

Emergency Department (ED) Coding

Emergency department (ED) codes represent services rendered in the ED and are reported with CPT codes 99281–99285. Although all three components of the E/M guidelines (HPI, examination, and MDM) are required to report these codes, CMS has acknowledged that the ED CPT codes do not adequately reflect the intensity of the patient's condition and the hospital resources that were required to treat and/or diagnose it. Therefore, CMS recommends that hospitals establish their own internal guidelines to report ED CPT codes that adequately describe their resource consumption while still following the intent of the CPT code descriptor.

Accurate Inpatient Coding

Inpatient coding describes services rendered to patients who are admitted into a hospital setting. CPT codes 99221–99223 are used to report the initial encounter by the admitting physician. In order to report one of these three levels of codes, either the documentation must meet a detailed or comprehensive history and exam or a minimum requirement of 30 minutes is spent with the patient. Be aware that Medicare requires the admitting physician to append modifier AI on their charges to indicate their role as the principal physician. If the documentation does not meet either of these standards, or the encounter is for subsequent inpatient care, report services using CPT codes 99231–99233, which only require a problem-focused history and exam or a minimum requirement of 15 minutes spent with the patient. Coding professionals also need to be familiar with present-on-admission (POA) indicators, hospital-acquired conditions (HACs), and diagnosis-related groups (DRGs).

2021 AMA Guidelines for Office and Other Outpatient E/M

Beginning on January 1, 2021, the American Medical Association (AMA) will enact new guidelines that relate to the coding of office and other outpatient E/M codes. Perhaps the biggest change of the 2021 CPT code set is that new patient codes (99202–99205) will no longer require the three key components and the established patient codes (99211–99215) will no longer require two of the three key components. Instead, E/M leveling will be based on the severity of MDM or the total time spent by the provider, including face-to-face and non-face-to-face time. Although a medically appropriate history and examination should be obtained, it is no longer a driving force to level an E/M code. Additionally, CPT code 99201 has been dissolved completely and CPT code 99211 is still available but is tailored for use by clinical staff members under the supervision of a physician with no suggested time requirements.

CMS Guidelines for Global Surgery Coding and Billing

The global surgery coding and billing guidelines include reporting and reimbursement rules for surgeries, endoscopies, and other minor procedures in any medical setting. CMS has created three types of global surgical packages built on the duration of the postoperative period. For example, endoscopies and some minor procedures have a **zero-day** postoperative period. Other minor procedures have a **10-day** postoperative period following the day of the surgery. Any major procedure has a **90-day** postoperative period following the day of the surgery. Unless an unrelated illness occurs, postoperative visits within these designated timeframes are considered a necessary part of surgical care and additional payment is not given. To determine if a procedure has a postoperative period, enter the CPT code into the Medicare Physician Fee Schedule lookup tool found here: https://www.cms.gov/apps/physician-fee-schedule/overview.aspx. Note that "Show All Columns" must be selected in order to locate the "Global" column.

Documentation Requirements for Reporting Consultations

A consultation is an encounter that occurs when a primary treating physician requests the opinion or advice regarding the evaluation and/or management of a specific illness from another qualified physician or nonphysician practitioner. When deciding to report a consultation service code, bear in mind the following four elements: request, reason, report, and intent. A request for the consultation, usually in the form of a referral, must be documented, along with the reason for such a request. A written report of the consulting physician's findings and/or recommendation must be transmitted back to the primary treating physician. Finally, the intent of the service should be evaluated. If the consulting physician is assuming immediate care of the patient's condition or if the other three elements are not met, an outpatient or subsequent hospital care E/M code should be reported instead.

Importance of Adherence by All Coding Professionals to Same Coding Rules and Conventions

It is important for all coding professionals to adhere to the same coding rules and conventions when assigning ICD-10-CM and CPT codes for **consistency in data**. Coded data are reviewed not only for reimbursement purposes, but for researchers to track public health and for the government to measure quality and safety practices. These data are collected for present and future use. However, in order for the data to be reliable and accurate, the same coding rules and conventions need to be followed by everyone. When coders allow reimbursement to inappropriately influence code assignment, they could potentially be putting their physician or entity at risk for audits, fines, and negative publicity.

Official Sources of Coding Information

Although there is an abundance of coding information available through encoders, published books, and Internet articles, coding professionals must be aware of where the official sources of coding guidelines and conventions can be found. Currently, there are four organizations responsible for the official coding guidelines and conventions. Together, they are referred to as the cooperating parties, and they include the American Health Information Management Association (AHIMA), the American Hospital Association, CMS, and the National Center for Health Statistics. The official guidelines and conventions that they stipulate can be found in the Introduction sections of the CPT, ICD-10-CM, and HCPCS Level II manuals; however, each organization publishes individual resources to help its members understand the relevant coding advice. Additionally, the Medical Library Association has provided the following tool on how to locate reliable information on the internet: https://www.mlanet.org/resources/userguide.html.

CPT/HCPCS Modifiers

Modifiers

A modifier is a two-character, alphanumeric code that is appended to CPT and HCPCS Level II procedure codes. A modifier may be reported to provide the insurance carrier with additional information regarding the circumstances surrounding the encounter. The use of modifiers is heavily dependent on which procedure or equipment is being reported, to whom it is being reported, and from which place of service it is being reported. Being familiar with all modifiers and when to use them is imperative because failing to report them and/or doing so incorrectly may lead to claim rejections, improper payments, delayed payments, or denials.

Modifier 25

Modifier 25 is a CPT modifier that is appended on a "significant, separately identifiable E/M **service** by the same physician" on the same day of another procedure or service. When deciding whether to report modifier 25, search for evidence that would warrant a separately billed E/M code that is **unrelated** to the procedure or service rendered on the same day. For example, if an established patient receives a biopsy of a suspicious lesion during a preventative care visit, the preventative care service would be billed with modifier 25, followed by the procedure code for the biopsy CPT code. On the other hand, if the primary reason for the visit was the biopsy, but hypertension was also discussed and medication was issued, the procedure code for the biopsy would be reported, followed by an E/M code with modifier 25.

Modifier 24

Modifier 24 is a CPT modifier that is appended on an **unrelated E/M service** rendered by the same physician during the postoperative period. Different procedures have different **postoperative periods**, generally ranging from 0 to 90 days, so it is imperative to know the postoperative period of a procedure prior to reporting. For example, the postoperative period of a dilation and curettage for the treatment of a missed abortion (CPT code 59820) is 90 days. A patient who received this surgery is now seen by the same provider 6 weeks later for a medication refill to treat a sexually transmitted disease. An appropriate use of modifier 24 would be to bill an E/M code with the modifier to indicate that treatment was rendered for an unrelated illness within 90 days of a major surgery.

HCPCS Level II Modifier

An HCPCS Level II modifier is a two-digit alphabetical or alphanumerical code that is appended to CPT and HCPCS Level II procedure codes to provide the insurance carrier with additional information and/or the circumstances surrounding the encounter or issued medical equipment, which may be required by the carrier. For example, a physical therapist creates long-term treatment goals for a patient with Medicare and sends them to the referring doctor for review. If the referring doctor signs that document, indicating his or her approval of such goals, the physical therapist may append modifier GP to their services, indicating that a plan of care has been established. Without this modifier, the physical therapy services may be denied. Level II modifiers are maintained by CMS and can be found in Appendix 2 of the HCPCS Level II Expert manual or at CMS.gov. Type "HCPCS release & code sets" into the search bar, and an updated list can be accessed, which is maintained and released quarterly.

Modifier 51 and Modifier 59

Modifier 51 is used when **multiple procedures** (excluding E/M and rehabilitation services) are performed during the same session by the same provider. Keywords such as "a different procedure" or "separate from" are indicators of when modifier 51 should be appended to the secondary procedure code. Modifier 59 is used to describe a procedure that is independent of other non-E/M services performed during the same session by the same provider. Modifier 59 is also used when reporting services that are not normally rendered together. Remember that with both modifiers, it is inappropriate to append them to add-on codes (AOCs).

Modifier 52 and Modifier 53

Modifier 52 is used when the services rendered are **reduced** by the decision of the provider. Keywords such as "partial," "part of the procedure eliminated," and "not completed" are indicators that modifier 52 should be appended to the procedure code. For example, if the removal of an intrauterine device was attempted, but it was unsuccessful due to embedment in the endometrium, report code 58301-52. Modifier 53 is used when a procedure is **discontinued**, perhaps for the well-being of the patient. Keywords such as "terminated" and "aborted" should be mentioned in the provider's documentation. As a similar example, if the removal of an intrauterine device was attempted but aborted due to excessive bleeding, report code 58301-53.

Modifier 58 and Modifier 78

Modifier 58 is used for a **staged procedure** by the same physician during the postoperative period. This means that the secondary procedure, tertiary procedure, and so forth are all planned to take place during the 0-, 10-, or 90-day postoperative period of the first procedure. Modifier 78 is for an **unexpected** return to the operating room by the same physician during the postoperative period to address a complication that has developed as a result of the initial procedure. The physician should document specifically what the complication is. For example, if a patient requires additional surgery within the 90-day postoperative period of a knee replacement to treat an infection that has developed at the incision site, append modifier 78. It should be noted that the billing of a new procedure with the use of modifier 78 does not extend the original postoperative period.

Modifier 26 and HCPCS Level II Modifier TC

Modifier 26 is appended to a procedure code to indicate that only the professional component of the service was rendered. For example, if a provider only interprets the images of a bilateral screening mammography, report code 77067-26. Modifier TC is appended to a procedure code to indicate that only the technical component of the service was rendered. For example, if a facility only performs a bilateral screening mammography without interpretation, report code 77067-TC to request reimbursement for only the equipment use. When the provider who owns the equipment also interprets the results or is employed by the entity who owns the equipment, do not report the procedure with a modifier. Also note that modifiers 26 and TC are not to be used with E/M services because these inherently include only a professional component.

Modifiers That May Be Appended to Anesthesia Codes (00100–01999)

A **physical status modifier** is informational and is used to identify different levels of complexity associated with a patient's condition. These modifiers are useful tools to support medical necessity and range from P1 to P6. **HCPCS Level II modifiers** are also appended when reporting the level of medical supervision and direction given. These include AA and AD for an anesthesiologist and QY, QX, and QZ for a certified registered nurse anesthetist (CRNA). Additional modifiers would include QS and G8 or G9, which indicate that monitored anesthesia care (MAC) services were rendered, and GA, GX, GY, and GZ, which relate to liability. A detailed description of each modifier can be found in the table below.

Modifier	Description
P1	A normal, healthy patient
P2	A patient with mild systemic disease
P3	A patient with severe systemic disease
P4	A patient with severe systemic disease that is a constant threat to life
P5	A moribund patient who is not expected to survive without the operation
P6	A declared brain-dead patient whose organs are being removed for donor purposes
AA	Anesthesia services performed by the anesthesiologist
AD	Medical supervision by a physician: more than four concurrent anesthesia procedures
QX	CRNA service: with medical direction by a physician
QY	Medical direction of one CRNA by an anesthesiologist
QZ	CRNA service: without medical direction by a physician
QS	MAC
G8	MAC for a deep, complex, complicated, or markedly invasive surgical procedure
G9	MAC for a patient who has history of severe cardiopulmonary condition
GA	Waiver of liability issued as required by payer policy, individual care
GX	Notice of liability issued, voluntary under payer policy
GY	Item or service statutorily excluded, does not meet the definition of any Medicare benefit or, for non-Medicare insurers, is not a contract benefit
GZ	Item or service expected to be denied as not reasonable and necessary

Note: To stay up to date on the current list and descriptions of modifiers, reference CMS.gov for the quarterly release of information by Medicare.

Modifier 23

Modifier 23 is a CPT modifier used to describe "unusual anesthesia" services. An anesthesia service is considered unusual when it is appended on a procedure code that does not normally involve the use of anesthesia. Modifier 23 is only appended on surgical procedure codes, never on anesthesia codes 00100–01999. An example of an extraordinary circumstance may be any procedure that is performed on a pediatric patient. In this case, the age of the patient would deem anesthesia use to be necessary for a procedure during which it is normally not used. When reporting unusual anesthesia services, be sure to submit supporting documentation to the insurance carrier.

Sequencing Diagnoses and Procedures

Sequencing Multiple Injuries on Same and on Different Anatomical Sites

When multiple injuries occur at different anatomical sites, sequence each injury in order from most severe to least severe. For example, if a patient presents with a closed ulnar fracture and an open femur fracture, the open femur fracture would be sequenced first because it is considered more critical because an open fracture is one that penetrates the skin and requires immediate medical attention to prevent an infection from developing at the wound site. When multiple injuries occur at the same anatomical site, only code the injury with the highest severity. For example, if a patient has a first-degree burn and a third-degree burn on his right hand, only code the third-degree burn because a first-degree burn affects only the outer layer of the skin whereas a third-degree burn involves the deep layers of the skin.

Acute and Chronic Conditions

Acute conditions are typically sudden, severe, and last less than 1 month. Acute conditions include respiratory failure, myocardial infarctions, and viral hepatitis. On the other hand, **chronic conditions** have a much slower onset and require ongoing medical attention that could last 1 or more years. Chronic conditions include cancer, diabetes, heart disease, and kidney disease. If a patient is diagnosed with a condition that is acute and chronic, and the ICD-10-CM manual contains separate entries for each, sequence the acute condition first, followed by the chronic disease. For example, for a patient diagnosed with acute on chronic deep vein thrombosis of the right lower extremity, report ICD-10-CM code I82.401 (Acute embolism and thrombosis of unspecified deep veins of right lower extremity) as the primary diagnosis, followed by ICD-10-CM code I82.501 (Chronic embolism and thrombosis of unspecified deep veins of right lower extremity) as the secondary diagnosis.

Sequencing Encounters for HIV

When it comes to HIV, chapter-specific guidelines provide direction on proper coding techniques. For example, when a patient who has a confirmed medical history of HIV is seen for an HIV-related illness, the principal diagnosis should be B20 (HIV disease), followed by any additional codes that identify the manifestation(s). If in doubt as to whether an illness is HIV-related, the ICD-10-CM manual contains black "HIV" icons next to all diagnosis codes that are deemed related to the virus. On the other hand, some patients have tested positive for HIV, but they never experience symptoms. In these cases, diagnosis code Z21 (Asymptomatic HIV infection status) would be reported and listed after the body system chapters because it is usually only informative and not the sole reason for the encounter.

Sequelae

A **sequela** is a residual effect that is a direct result of an injury or illness that has been healed or cured. An example of a sequela may be a scar that forms on the skin after an acute burn has healed.

Unless the manifestation of the injury is included in the sequela diagnosis code, the ICD-10-CM code describing the manifestation should be sequenced first, followed by the code for the injury. In the same example, the ICD-10-CM code for the scar would be sequenced first, followed by the burn. Because residual effects can become apparent either immediately or many years later, there are no restrictions on when a sequela may be reported.

Malignancy

The ICD-10-CM code representing the particular malignancy should be the principal diagnosis when the patient is receiving treatment directly for the malignancy, except if the reason for the encounter is for the administration of chemotherapy, immunotherapy, or external beam radiation therapy. Additionally, if the reason for the encounter is to treat anemia or another complication associated with a malignancy, the malignancy should again be the principal diagnosis, followed by the associated complication diagnosis. However, if the reason for the encounter is to treat a secondary site of metastasis only, the secondary site should be coded as the principal diagnosis. To ensure proper coding of a malignancy, coding professionals should review the chapter-specific guidelines in the ICD-10-CM manual prior to reporting.

Sequencing Obstetric Patients

When reporting diagnoses for an obstetric patient, coders should review the specific guidelines set forth in Chapter 15 relating to pregnancy, childbirth, and postpartum. When reporting illnesses and/or injuries of an individual who is pregnant, a code should be selected from the range O00–O9A, followed by additional codes from other chapters when applicable. For example, if an obstetric patient is seen to discuss the management of her type I diabetes, O24.01 (Pre-existing type 1 diabetes mellitus, in pregnancy) should be sequenced first, followed by E10.9 (Type 1 diabetes mellitus without complications). Reporting should always end with a Z3A. code, indicating the gestational age of the fetus. An exception to this rule occurs when a provider specifically states in their documentation that a condition being treated is not affecting the pregnancy. In that case, use the appropriate disease illness or injury code found outside of Chapter 15, followed by Z33.1 (Pregnant state, incidental).

Discerning Which Additional Diagnoses Should Be Reported

When multiple diagnoses are listed in a medical record, ICD-10-CM guidelines stipulate that only illnesses that affect the patient's care should be reported on the claim. That means that the condition may require additional clinical evaluation, therapeutic treatment, diagnostic procedures, an extended hospital stay length, and/or increased nursing care or monitoring. Similarly, when a physician documents that a patient has a personal or family history of an illness and/or injury, a Z code may be reported as a secondary code if it influences the current care or treatment.

Selection and Sequencing of Diagnoses

Example Medical Record

The patient presented with increased lower extremity edema and was noted to have significant anasarca. The patient has a history of acute on chronic systolic heart failure, which I believe is the cause. The patient's blood pressure was noted to be elevated, with a history of hypertension. Due to the patient's stage II chronic kidney disease (CKD), creatinine levels were obtained.

The first step is to search for "Failure" in the ICD-10-CM index because it seems that the heart failure is the underlying illness for the encounter. Follow it through to "Heart," "Systolic," "Acute," and then "And chronic I50.23." An associated note appears with diagnosis code I50.23, to code I11.0, Heart failure due to hypertension, or I13.-, Heart failure due to hypertension with chronic kidney disease, first. Although the physician does not explicitly state that the heart failure is "due to" hypertension or that the patient has hypertension "with" CKD, chapter-specific guidelines instruct coders to assume that a causal relationship exists between these conditions, unless the physician documents that they are unrelated. Therefore, the appropriate code selection would be I13.0, Hypertensive heart and chronic kidney disease with heart failure and stages 1 through 4 chronic kidney disease. Another note appears to use an additional code to identify the stage of CKD, which can be reflected with N18.2, Chronic kidney disease, stage 2. The final diagnosis, anasarca, literally meaning generalized edema, is a symptom that is not coded because a definitive diagnosis of heart failure exists. Thus, the appropriate way to report this encounter is I13.0, I50.23, and N18.2.

Selection and Sequencing of Procedures

Example Medical Record

The physician suspects malignancy and decides to remove two lesions from the patient's back to confirm. The first lesion has a diameter of 0.5 cm, and the excised diameter is 1.0 cm. The second lesion has a diameter of 0.3 cm, and the excised diameter is 1.5 cm.

Based on the documentation, the primary reason for the visit is the excision of lesions. Locate the root procedure "Excision" in the index of the CPT manual. The excision procedures are separated by anatomy. Next, select "Skin." Under this subheading, a coding professional can either select whether the procedure was for the removal of malignant or benign lesions. Without a pathology report to confirm malignancy, CPT guidelines state that the excision code assumes that the lesion is benign, leading a coder to CPT codes 11400–11471. Review of these codes leads to the selection of 11401 (Excision, benign lesion including margins, except skin tag, trunk; excised diameter 0.6 to 1.0 cm) and 11402 (Excision, benign lesion including margins, except skin tag, trunk; excised diameter 1.1 to 2.0 cm). CPT code 11402 would be listed first because the highest dollar value code takes priority in sequencing, followed by CPT code 11401 with modifier 59 to indicate an additional and separate procedure.

Present-on-Admission (POA) Guidelines

POA Guidelines

In 2007, the United States government implemented **present-on-admission** (POA) guidelines as a way to reduce unnecessary costs incurred to the Medicare program. Under these guidelines, general acute-care hospitals and facilities became responsible for differentiating illnesses and/or injuries that an individual presented with upon their admission from those that developed later during their inpatient stay. General acute-care hospitals and facilities differentiate these conditions by means of one of five indicators that can be attached to the principal and secondary diagnoses on an electronic or paper claim.

POA Indicators

The following are the five POA indicators used by acute-care hospitals and facilities:

POA Indicator	Description
Y	Yes — The diagnosis was present at the time of inpatient admission; CMS will pay.
N	No — The diagnosis was not present at the time of inpatient admission; CMS will not pay.
U	Unknown — The documentation is insufficient to determine if the condition is POA; CMS will not pay.

POA Indicator	Description
W	Clinically undetermined — The provider is unable to clinically determine whether the condition was POA or not; CMS will pay.
1	Unreported/Not used — Exempt from POA reporting; CMS will not pay.

Benefits of POA Guidelines

CMS is authorized to make or adjust payments to hospitals and facilities based on the POA indicators that they are provided with. In doing so, their aim is to reduce unnecessary costs due to errors, injuries, and infections that could have been prevented by the healthcare staff. For example, if an infection was reported as not present at the time of admission, Medicare is not responsible for the payment of the services that were subsequently required to treat and cure the infection during an individual's inpatient stay. As a result, hospitals and facilities are compelled to provide better care to their patients from the beginning of their treatment plans.

Example of When POA Indicator Y Should Be Reported

POA indicator Y is used when an illness or injury is present at the time of an admission. Although some diagnoses are obviously present prior to admission — such as a history of hypertension, diabetes mellitus, or asthma — others must be inferred from the documentation. For example, a patient admitted for a diagnostic workup of a fever and difficulty breathing has a discharge note revealing pneumonia. Although the pneumonia was not explicitly stated at the time of admission, the individual's symptoms provide a clear picture that the illness existed and was POA. Additionally, this same rule applies toward possible, probable, suspected, and ruled-out diagnoses and for conditions that develop during an outpatient encounter.

Example of When POA Indicator N Should Be Reported

POA indicator N is used when an illness or injury is not present at the time of an admission but develops during an individual's inpatient stay. Illnesses that are usually not present at the time of an admission would include postoperative infections and pressure ulcers, also known as bedsores. However, also included in this category may be acute exacerbations of chronic illnesses and obstetric conditions. For example, if a patient with a history of chronic obstructive pulmonary disorder (COPD) develops a flare-up after they are admitted, the POA indicator associated with the COPD diagnosis code would be N. A second example of the appropriate use of the POA indicator N may be if a laceration occurred during the delivery of a fetus.

POA Indicator U vs. POA Indicator W

POA indicator U is used when the documentation is insufficient to determine if the condition was POA. This can occur when a provider does not obtain a detailed history intake that includes signs and symptoms, thus making it difficult to understand the etiology of a disease and its manifestation timeline. **POA indicator W** is used when the provider has sufficiently documented the course of treatment and testing but cannot clinically determine when the condition was established. For example, if a breast abscess is discovered when an obstetric patient attempts to breastfeed after the delivery of her child, W would be the appropriate POA indicator to report with the breast abscess diagnosis code.

Assigning Accurate POA Indicators

POA indicators play a large role in the revenue cycle. Repeated attempts to submit claims with an associated POA indicator U, for example, may lead to Medicare denials and requests for audits, ultimately resulting in a major loss of revenue for a hospital or facility. Therefore, if a coding professional cannot determine the presence of a condition at the time of admission, the provider should be queried for clarification. Additionally, because a physician is legally accountable for establishing a patient's diagnosis, assigning the most accurate POA indicator is imperative if the case might ever be examined in a courtroom.

Entities and Diagnoses Exempt from POA Guidelines

The POA guidelines encompass only acute general care hospitals and facilities. Therefore, entities such as long-term-care hospitals, children's inpatient facilities, cancer hospitals, inpatient psychiatric hospitals, and inpatient rehabilitation facilities are all exempt from reporting POA indicators. CMS also deems certain medical diagnoses as exempt from this provision as well. For example, illnesses arising from an intracerebral hemorrhage, such as monoplegia, dysphagia, and other sequelae, are common and may occur sometime after a patient is admitted. Because these conditions are usually not preventable, hospitals are not held financially responsible. A complete list of exempt diagnosis codes for the current fiscal year can be viewed at https://www.cms.gov/Medicare/Medicare-Fee-for-Service-Payment/HospitalAcqCond/Coding.

Ways Hospitals Can Improve Accuracy of POA Coding

Though its institution has been in place for well over a decade, a recent study reports that the assignment of accurate POA indicators remains problematic for many hospitals across the country. Although there are multiple factors to consider, the most obvious reason for the discrepancies could be variations in coding practices and a shortage of trained coding personnel. To counteract these factors and improve the accuracy of POA coding, hospitals may consider initiating screening protocols, such as internal audits, prior to any code-related submissions in order to identify errors and suggest improvement strategies. Hospitals may also consider obtaining and promoting guidelines for POA designations among their staff to educate them on proper coding techniques. By being proactive in these ways, a hospital can ensure high-quality care and optimal reimbursement rates.

POA Guidelines for Combination Codes

A combination code is a single ICD-10-CM code that can encompass two diagnoses or a single diagnosis with an associated manifestation or complication. An example of a combination code would be ICD-10-CM code E11.52, Type 2 diabetes mellitus with diabetic gangrene. In this case, if the type 2 diabetes mellitus and gangrene — or symptoms of these illnesses — were present prior to admission, the POA indicator would be Y. On the other hand, if the patient only presented with one disease, in this case type 2 diabetes mellitus, and developed an associated complication after the admission, the POA indicator would be N.

Coding Edits

Role of the NCCI

The National Correct Coding Initiative (NCCI) was created in 1994 by CMS to **prevent incorrect payments** due to **improper coding**. Improper coding includes unbundled procedure codes, as well as failing to append a modifier on some services that are performed together. The NCCI policy manual is a useful tool to help providers, suppliers, and hospitals identify errors in their billing practices and to help prevent payment denials and carrier-specific audits. The NCCI policy manual is updated quarterly by CMS and can be found at https://www.cms.gov/Medicare/Coding/NationalCorrectCodInitEd.

NCCI Edits

An NCCI edit is a pair of procedures, services, medicines, and/or durable medical equipment that is normally not separately reportable by the same provider and/or supplier for one date of service; however, it may be separately reportable under certain circumstances and with the appropriate modifier. CMS has created these edits to help aid providers combat improper coding. These edits serve to inform both parties whether two codes may be billed together without a coding modifier, with a modifier, or in some cases, that under no circumstance should these two CPT/HCPCS codes be billed together.

Edits Created by the NCCI

CMS has created three types of edits in its NCCI policy manual to help providers combat improper coding. The first is known as a **medically unlikely edit (MUE)**. MUEs identify the maximum number of units that may be reported for a CPT/HCPCS code that relate to an individual patient. The second type of edit is called a **procedure-to-procedure (PTP)** edit. This type of edit alerts the provider of two procedures that are mutually exclusive of each other. In other words, it would be unreasonable to have performed these two procedures and/or services during the same session. The third edit is an **add-on code (AOC),** which is used when a service and/or procedure follows another primary CPT/HCPCS code.

Interpreting the NCCI Policy Manual Format

The NCCI policy manual is designed so that every possible CPT/HCPCS code combination being submitted by the same provider on the same date of service is presented in columns. **Column one** contains the primary or major procedure or service that was performed, and **column two** contains the secondary or lesser procedure/service. Following the code combination will be one of these three modifiers: **0, 1, or 9**. These modifiers reflect proper coding techniques. The modifier "0" means that the combination of codes should never, under any circumstance, be reported together; "1" means that the codes may be reported together with the use of a coding modifier; and "9" means that codes in the combination are reportable on their own and that they do not require a coding modifier. The policy also contains the **effective date** of all edits and, where applicable, the **deletion date** of an edit.

MUE

A medically unlikely edit (MUE) factors in human anatomy, prescription instructions, and code descriptions to decide the maximum number of units that may be reported for a CPT/HCPCS code. For example, as of April 1, 2020, the maximum number of units that may be reported for CPT code 44960 (Appendectomy; for ruptured appendix with abscess or generalized peritonitis) is one. Simply put, because the human body only contains one appendix, it would be unreasonable for the procedure to be performed more than once. As a second example, CPT code 46940 (Curettage or cautery of anal fissure, including dilation of anal sphincter; initial) has a maximum allowable of one unit. This is due to the fact that there can only ever be one "initial" procedure. It is important to note that not all CPT/HCPCS codes will have an MUE.

PTP Edit

A procedure-to-procedure (PTP) edit factors in CPT manual and CMS coding instructions, definitions, and standards of practice to decide which CPT/HCPCS codes would be considered inclusive to another. For example, as of July 1, 2020, CPT code 99221 in column one (Initial hospital care, per day, for the evaluation and management of a patient) and CPT code 99281 in column two (Emergency department visit for the evaluation and management of a patient) contain the modifier 0, indicating that under no circumstance can these procedures be reported together. This decision is based on CPT coding instructions, which state that when a provider admits a patient, all services that were rendered by that provider on that day would be considered inclusive to the admission code (99221).

AOC Edit

An add-on code (AOC) edit provides an acceptable list of primary CPT/HCPCS codes that may be paired with a specific AOC. Oftentimes, the CPT manual provides this information, but in some cases, it does not list every appropriate primary CPT/HCPCS code that pairs with an AOC. For example, as of April 1, 2020, add-on CPT code 69990 (Microsurgical techniques, requiring use of operating microscope) may be reported in conjunction with primary CPT code 61304 (Craniectomy or craniotomy, exploratory; supratentorial). This edit is not found in the CPT manual; rather, it is in the list of AOC edits provided by CMS. It should also be noted that just because the CMS and CPT manuals state that an AOC is reportable, this does not ensure payment. Payment of a primary procedure must be considered payable before payment of an AOC is issued.

Dangers of Not Complying with the NCCI

Because the NCCI was created to prevent incorrect payments due to improper coding, not following its guidelines may pose significant consequences. These include, but are not limited to, claim **rejections**, claim **denials**, payment **recoupments**, carrier-specific **audits**, and even claims of **abuse** or **fraud**. The best way to prevent improper coding is to identify and understand the root causes of denials, receive proper training and education on the latest coding updates, and to implement a proactive strategy plan to resolve improper coding patterns and trends, such as employing an auditor to review a case before it is sent to an insurance carrier.

Determining If CPT Code 97530 Is Reportable with CPT Code 97164 Using the NCCI Policy Manual

For the most up-to-date NCCI edits, visit the NCCI edits page of the Medicare website: https://www.cms.gov/Medicare/Coding/NationalCorrectCodInitEd. Because only one unit of each is being billed, and neither one is considered an AOC, select the PTP edits link. Search for CPT code 97530 (Therapeutic activities, direct patient contact by the provider, each 15 minutes) in column one, followed by CPT code 97164 (Re-evaluation of physical therapy established plan of care) in column two. The edit modifier listed is "1," indicating that a modifier is required to report these services together. CMS has deemed that unless a change has occurred in the patient's status that deems a re-evaluation service medically necessary, CPT 97164 should not be routinely reported; however, when it should be reported, the edits may be bypassed with modifier 59.

Reimbursement Classifications

Out-of-Pocket Expenses

Out-of-pocket expenses are the costs of medical care that are not covered by a federal or commercial health insurance plan. Out-of-pocket expenses include deductibles, copayments, and coinsurances. A **deductible** is the amount that an individual must pay for covered services prior to a health insurance plan paying. For example, most Medicare Part B plans require a person to first pay a $200 deductible into any healthcare services that they receive. After a deductible has been met, a patient may be required to pay a copayment or coinsurance. A **copayment** is a fixed amount that a person has to pay to receive certain health services, such as $20 for each visit to a specialist. A **coinsurance** is a percentage that a person pays for covered healthcare services. For example, a 20% coinsurance payment on a $100 office visit would cause an individual to pay $20 and his or her health insurance plan to pay the remaining $80.

DRGs

Prior to 1982, hospitals were paid on each charge they submitted, leading to extended hospital stays and unnecessary costs to the government. In order to control the costs of health care and encourage hospitals to provide the most efficient care, Medicare and other health insurance plans have adopted diagnostic related groups (DRGs). **DRGs** refer to a classification system that factors the age, gender, diagnosis, and procedures performed during a patient's inpatient hospital stay to determine how much the hospital should be paid. Although the base rate of a DRG is adjusted by location and cost of living, the reimbursement rates are considered standardized and fixed.

Negative Impact on Health Care and Medicare's Efforts to Overcome It

Although the framework to standardize hospital reimbursement was intended to control healthcare costs and encourage efficient care, the implementation of DRGs has had its own set of challenges. One challenge is that the DRG payment system has created a financial incentive for hospitals to discharge their patients. That is, in order to make a profit, hospitals have discharged patients before they are healthy enough to return home, which has resulted in **readmissions**. To counteract that, Medicare has rules in place to penalize a hospital if a readmission occurs within 30 days of the original discharge date and involves the same diagnosis.

HCCs

The **hierarchical condition categories (HCCs)** were established in 2004 as a way to assign a risk adjustment factor (RAF) score to certain diagnosis codes. Currently, of the 70,000+ ICD-10-CM codes, approximately 9,500 are associated to 1 of the 79 HCCs. The RAF score is used by health insurance plans to predict payment costs and resource consumption of specific patient populations over time. For example, patients with chronic conditions are considered to be a higher risk population due to the need for continued treatment and monitoring. In order to ensure maximum reimbursement and correct patient care and outcomes, providers and coding professionals should be educated on the importance of documenting chronic conditions. For a complete list of ICD-10-CM codes associated with HCCs, visit https://www.cms.gov/Medicare/Health-Plans/MedicareAdvtgSpecRateStats/Risk-Adjustors.

Outcome and Assessment Information Set

The home health **Outcome and Assessment Information Set** is a quality measurement tool that is used to report and improve the quality of care delivered to Medicare and Medicaid patients in the home health setting. The data collected include observation, interviews with the patient and other associated healthcare providers, and a review of the related medical records. Based on this information, a home health agency will develop and implement a quality improvement plan. Assessments are performed at the start of care followed by a reassessment every 60 days, and again at either the death, discharge, or transfer of the patient to an inpatient facility. A home health agency is required to submit the data to CMS within 30 days of their collection.

Resource-Based Relative Value Scales

The **resource-based relative value scale** is a physician payment system adopted by CMS and other health insurance plans. Payments are calculated by combining the cost of the physician's work, practice expense, and professional liability insurance. The value is then multiplied by a conversion factor and adjusted based on the geographic location where the services were rendered, known as the geographic practice cost index. The resulting amount is known as a fee schedule payment. Understanding Medicare's resource-based relative value scales can help a practice to establish physician charges and calculate Medicare payments. For help with a fee schedule payment search, Medicare has provided the following lookup tool: https://www.cms.gov/apps/physician-fee-schedule/overview.aspx.

Managed Care Plans

A **managed care plan** describes a type of health insurance plan that organizes the provision, quality, and cost of care for its members. Usually, that includes selecting a primary care physician who will manage a member's care and, if medically necessary, issue a referral to another medical specialist. This is done in an effort to promote preventative health care (getting vaccinated, regular exercise, a healthy diet) and preventing reactive treatment. Although some health insurance plans issue payments to their members for health services, a managed care plan pays the provider directly, less the cost of any out-of-pocket expenses that the patient is responsible for.

Out-of-Network and In-Network Benefits

In-network means that a physician or entity has an agreement with a health insurance plan to provide medical services at a negotiated rate. It is usually more advantageous for a member to be treated by a physician or entity within their health insurance plan's network. **Out-of-network** means that a physician or entity does not have an agreement with a health insurance plan. The charges incurred from receiving treatment from a physician or entity not covered in the network is usually much higher than if a person were to receive treatment from an in-network physician. Coding professionals should have knowledge of which health insurance plans their physician or entity is in network with to prevent denials and exorbitant patient costs.

Various Plans

The Healthy Humans Plus Plan offers its members in- and out-of-network benefits. Although the patient has a $0 copayment, they are subject to their in- and out-of-network deductibles. The in-network deductible for an individual under this plan is $1,600, and the out-of-network deductible is $2,375. This plan has benefits for inpatient professional services, such as radiology and anesthesiology. If a member were to receive these services by an in-network physician, the health insurance plan pays 75% of the cost incurred after the deductible is met. This means that if the services cost $3,000, the member would have to pay their $1,600 deductible, plus the remaining 25%. However, if the member were to receive these services from an out-of-network physician, the health insurance plan pays only 55% of the cost incurred after the deductible is met. In this scenario, the member would be responsible for their $2,275 deductible, plus the remaining 45%. There is no cost incurred on the member when/if they choose to see their primary care physician.

Language Associated with Reimbursement

Medical professionals and entities can request reimbursement for healthcare services that they have rendered by submitting an **electronic or paper claim** to a beneficiary's health insurance plan. These claims contain details of the encounter in the form of CPT and ICD-10-CM codes, with the associated charges. Once the health insurance plan has received and reviewed the claim — usually within 30 days — they will respond by sending a **remittance advice notice** to the medical professional or entity where services were rendered and an **explanation of benefits** to the beneficiary. These documents identify the **allowable amount**, or how much the insurance has approved to pay; the **beneficiary responsibility** in the form of a copayment, deductible, or coinsurance; and the reasons for any charges that were **denied** or not paid.

Internal Appeal Letter

When a health insurance plan denies payment for healthcare services already rendered, an individual can send an appeal letter requesting them to reconsider their decision. An appeal letter can request the reconsideration of any denial that involves medical judgment, experimental or investigational treatment, and/or coverage issues in which the health insurance plan provided incomplete or false information of the beneficiary. The first step to creating an appeal letter is to understand the reason for denial and collect supporting evidence to counteract it. For example, if the reason for denial is that the treatment is considered experimental, search for recent studies that confirm positive outcomes using a similar plan of care. When writing the appeal letter, keep the content concise, factual, and related to the denial reason. When appropriate, include supporting evidence, official coding conventions and guidelines, and/or medical reports. Additionally, coding professionals and physicians should include their credentials to show the health insurance plan who is involved in the appeal process. In general, health insurance plans typically respond to an appeal within 30 days.

Requesting External Reviews

If a physician or coding professional feels that an internal appeal has been denied incorrectly, an external review performed by the state or the Department of Health and Human Services (HHS) may be requested within 4 months of the denial notice. Typically, the remittance advice will provide the contact information for whom an external review should be requested through. Once an external review request has been received, the turnaround time can be as soon as 24 hours, but it should be no later than 45 days. When a decision has been rendered, the health insurance plan is required by law to accept that decision. For more details on internal appeals and external reviews, visit https://www.hhs.gov/healthcare/about-the-law/cancellations-and-appeals/appealing-health-plan-decisions/index.html.

ABN

An **advance beneficiary notice of noncoverage (ABN)** is a notice given by physicians, suppliers, religious nonmedical healthcare institutions, and home health agencies to beneficiaries when a service is expected to be denied by Medicare Parts A or B. If a beneficiary chooses to sign the ABN notice, they are accepting financial liability for any services rendered that are denied. Medicare requires the ABN to be given to the beneficiary far enough in advance for them to review their medical options and make an informed decision. This form is not for use in emergent or urgent healthcare situations. To download an ABN form from CMS, visit http://www.cms.gov/Medicare/Medicare-General-Information/BNI/ABN.html.

OPPS

The hospital Outpatient Prospective Payment System (OPPS) was developed in 2000 as a reimbursement method for Medicare patients receiving **outpatient services**, with the exception of laboratory, outpatient therapy, and mammography services, **in a hospital setting**. For each fiscal year, the OPPS establishes rates of payment in order to promote the predictability of payment, promote consistency, and encourage efficient and quality care. If a claim submitted is determined to be payable under the OPPS, a payment status indicator is assigned to indicate which reimbursement methodology should be used, such as Ambulatory Payment Classifications, fee schedule, or reasonable cost. For additional information on the OPPS or to review annual updates, visit https://www.cms.gov/Medicare/Medicare-Fee-for-Service-Payment/HospitalOutpatientPPS.

Coding Professional's Role in Medical Reimbursement

A coding professional has a direct role in medical reimbursement. As they review a medical record, ICD-10-CM, CPT, and HCPCS codes are assigned based on the documented clinical information provided. This reported information is then used by health insurance plans, researchers, and government agencies who determine the cost benefits and limitations of a beneficiary. For example, if the payment methodology is DRG, Medicare examines the principal diagnosis code to determine a fixed payment for the care provided. On the other hand, if the reported information is not accurate, physicians and healthcare organizations face potential revenue losses, denials, or audits.

Revenue Cycle Management

According to the AMA, the revenue cycle refers to the "business side" of a practice — from patient intake and eligibility to the receival of health insurance plan and patient payments. In order for a revenue cycle to operate in an efficient manner, all clinical and nonclinical staff members must work together to collect, enter, and report the most accurate patient encounter information. Additionally, when services are denied payment, an effective denial team will work to rectify the issue in a timely manner. If any part of the revenue cycle management is out of sync or deficient, a healthcare practice faces potential revenue losses that could last years. Revenue cycle management is necessary if a physician wishes to create an efficient and sustainable healthcare practice.

Abstracting Pertinent Data

Medical Record Layout

Although documentation methods vary for each physician, the medical record will generally begin with the patient's chief complaint, which is the primary reason for the encounter. Following that would be a patient's past, social, and family history. This information may or may not be contained in separate tabs in an electronic medical record. Next may be an ROS, in which the patient has the opportunity to confirm or deny signs and symptoms pertaining to their different body systems. Next is a physical exam, usually focused around the patient's chief complaint. Once the physician has collected an intake from the patient and examined the patient, he or she can make a diagnosis and a plan of how to address the patient's concerns.

Verbiage Associated with Diagnosis

At times, a physician may simply list multiple conditions in the assessment without fully addressing them throughout the rest of the medical record. Unless the documentation can provide evidence of how a condition is monitored, evaluated, assessed, or treated, it should never be captured. On the other hand, coding professionals should look for certain verbiage that supports the reporting of any condition listed in the assessment. For example, if diabetes is documented, a simple notation such as "A1C improved, recheck glucose in 1 month" or "continue medication" is sufficient. Another example may be if a patient is obese. If the physician documents that "exercise was encouraged and diet was discussed," that is also enough supporting evidence to capture the diagnosis.

Common Errors with Data Abstraction

Coding professionals should be wary of reporting multiple chronic conditions simply because a physician has listed them in an assessment. A coding professional would not know if chronic conditions are current anymore, unless there is a plan of care attached to the condition. Additionally, there may be conflicting documentation in the medical chart for a single encounter. For example, a physician may document in the HPI that a diabetic patient has no illness-related complications but also reports diabetes with polyneuropathy in the assessment. In that case, the physician should be queried for clarification. Physicians and coding staff should be educated on the documentation requirements surrounding data abstraction.

Effect of Data Abstraction on Reimbursement

When reporting diagnosis codes, **specificity** is the key to maximizing reimbursement. For example, a physician may document that a patient suffers from CKD, a disease process that affects the body in different stages. The RAF score for CKD without a specified stage is 0. However, the RAF score for

CKD stages 4 and 5 is 0.237, and it is 0.422 for end-stage renal disease. The more specific and severe a condition is, the higher the RAF score, and the higher reimbursement will be. On the other hand, when the RAF score is reduced, so is the reimbursement.

Conditions and Comorbidities

Comorbidity

A comorbidity occurs when a patient has two or more unrelated diseases or disorders occurring at the same time. An example of a comorbidity may be a patient who suffers from a bone fracture and type II diabetes. Because a physician would need to consider both conditions when creating a treatment plan, both should be coded. The chief complaint or reason for the encounter should be coded as the primary diagnosis, the concurring disease should be reported as secondary, and so on. In the same scenario, if the patient were being treated by an orthopedist, the bone fracture would be coded as primary and the secondary code would be type II diabetes.

Not Reporting Comorbidities

When a patient has two or more unrelated diseases or disorders occurring at the same time, but the physician does not consider, inquire about, and/or treat the comorbid condition(s), only the chief complaint or reason for the encounter would be reported. For example, a patient with a history of severe asthma is seen by a dermatologist to have a skin lesion excised. The dermatologist removes the skin lesion but does not ask about the patient's severe asthma. In this scenario, even though the severe asthma is documented in the patient's medical record, it would not be a reported condition because it has no effect on the current care or treatment.

Complications Caused by Comorbidities

According to the Centers for Disease Control and Prevention, at least 1.7 million adults in America develop sepsis from underlying conditions each year, with the majority of them being readmitted into the hospital within 30 days. This is because many people carry other serious chronic conditions that can be difficult to manage after developing sepsis, even when it has resolved. For example, if a diabetic patient suffered from sepsis, their blood glucose levels may be harder to manage, leading to hyperglycemia, chronic wounds, and infections that the body cannot fight off. Another example is patients with COPD. Often, a history of sepsis leads to acute exacerbations and pneumonia, leading to the recurrence of sepsis, or even death.

Higher Risks Associated with Presence of Multiple Comorbidities in Heart Failure

When it comes to heart failure, patients are likely to develop additional cardiovascular and noncardiovascular comorbidities. According to a 2003 study published in the *Journal of the American College of Cardiology*, patients who suffer from heart failure often have four or more comorbidities. Among these include illnesses such as hypertension, ischemic heart disease, atrial fibrillation or flutter, valve disease, stroke, COPD, diabetes, renal disease, and anemia. The presence of these multiple comorbidities signals a higher risk patient group due to the increased complexity of medical management and the increased level of clinical decision making. Comorbid conditions become risk factors to future health deterioration and jeopardize positive patient outcomes.

Optimizing Patient Outcomes Related to Comorbidities

In order to optimize patient outcomes, a physician should be aware of the associated comorbidities surrounding any illness or disease. By having a thorough knowledge of the potential health issues that a patient may experience, physicians will be better able to identify symptoms and begin treatment at an early stage of the disease process. Physicians should also maintain good communication with other healthcare professionals involved in a patient's care. It is also recommended that medication and dosages should be reviewed regularly and adjusted when necessary, such as when the patient experiences a comorbidity.

Relationship Between Comorbidities and Coding

Researchers and health insurance plans rely heavily on the reported comorbidity data to predict risk and the associated healthcare costs. For example, researchers have been able to discern from coded data that hypertension is commonly associated with Alzheimer's disease and dementia, resulting in a push for frequent follow-up care. Additionally, Medicare has been able to estimate the cost that a beneficiary will incur on the government based on their medical history. However, in order for their predictions to be accurate, the coded data must be reliable. A coding professional must thoroughly examine the entire medical record to understand which comorbidities should be captured and how they should be reported.

Coding Documentation

Assigning Diagnosis and Procedure Codes

Assigning Diagnosis and Procedure Codes

Example Encounter

A 72-year-old patient is admitted due to atrial fibrillation. A comprehensive electrophysiology study is completed with fluoroscopic guidance, followed by a cardiac catheter ablation during the same procedure. The procedure took 22 minutes, and the patient was moderately sedated.

CPT codes: 93656, 99152

ICD-10-CM code: I48.91

Step 1: Locate the "Electrophysiology" procedure in the CPT manual index, leading to 93619–93620, 93653–93654, and 93656. After a review of each description, only CPT code 93656 describes a comprehensive electrophysiology study with a cardiac ablation of atrial fibrillation in the same session. Additionally, the added note attached to the code advises that if moderate sedation was used, it should be reported with CPT codes 99151–99153. Only CPT code 99152 fits the patient's age and the time requirement of the code.

Step 2: Locate "Fibrillation" in the ICD-10-CM manual index because this is the primary reason for the encounter.

Step 3: Select "Atrial." Because the documentation does not specify if the condition is chronic or persistent, the selection should be unspecified.

Example Encounter

A 15-year-old patient is being treated for obstructive sleep apnea and adenoid tissue hypertrophy. After being placed under general anesthesia, a dental mirror is placed in the oropharynx to allow visualization of the nasopharynx. Suction electrocautery is used to remove the adenoid tissue that regrew after the initial adenoidectomy. Attention is then turned to the tonsils. The plane of tissue between the tonsillar capsule and the underlying muscles is cauterized, and the tonsils are removed. Bleeding is controlled by silver nitrate and gauze packing. The procedure is completed without complications, and the patient is discharged to recovery.

CPT code: 42821

ICD-10-CM codes: J35.2, G47.33

Step 1: Understand that an adenoidectomy and a tonsillectomy were performed in this surgical encounter. A primary adenoidectomy refers to the initial removal of the adenoid, whereas a secondary adenoidectomy occurs when adenoid tissue that was once removed has grown back.

Step 2: Locate "Adenoidectomy" in the CPT manual index.

Step 3: Select "Secondary" and "With tonsillectomy." When an adenoidectomy and tonsillectomy are performed during the same session for a patient 12 years old and older, they are bundled into CPT code 42821.

Step 4: Locate "Hypertrophy" in the ICD-10-CM manual index.

Step 5: Select "Adenoids" and review ICD-10-CM code J35.2.

Step 6: Locate "Sleep" in the ICD-10-CM manual index.

Step 7: Select "Obstructive" and review ICD-10-CM code G47.33. ICD-10-CM guidelines state that when two conditions meet the definition for principal diagnosis, either one may be sequenced first.

Example Encounter

An 8-year-old female patient is seen by her pediatrician in the office for an allergic reaction to a bee sting. The pediatrician administers 0.3 mg of epinephrine through an intramuscular injection.

CPT codes: 96372, J0171x3

ICD-10-CM code: T63.441A

Step 1: Locate "Injection" in the CPT manual index.

Step 2: Select "Intramuscular" and review CPT code 96372. Because this CPT code includes an inherent E/M component, no separate office visit is reported. Additionally, because the epinephrine came directly from the physician, this, too, should be coded.

Step 3: Locate the "Table of Common Drugs" in the HCPCS manual.

Step 4: Locate "Epinephrine." Review HCPCS code J0171, considering that the documentation reflects a dosage of 0.3 mg.

Step 5: Locate "Venom" in the "Table of Drugs and Chemicals" in the ICD-10-CM manual.

Step 6: Select "Bee" and review ICD-10-CM code T63.441. The seventh character, A, should be added to indicate active treatment.

Example Encounter

A 92-year-old female patient with Medicare Part A coverage receives ongoing hospice care due to dementia. She goes to an orthopedic office to receive closed treatment of a left hip dislocation following a fall. No anesthesia was used.

CPT code: 27250-GW

ICD-10-CM codes: S73.002A, W19.XXXA

Step 1: Locate "Hip joint" in the CPT manual index.

Step 2: Select "Dislocation" and review CPT code 27250. Modifier GW should be added to patients receiving hospice because it indicates to Medicare that services are being rendered that are unrelated to their terminal illness. An inherent E/M component is included, so an additional office visit should not be reported.

Step 3: Locate "Dislocation" in the ICD-10-CM manual index.

Step 4: Select "Hip," and choose the appropriate left side, followed by the seventh character, A, to indicate active treatment.

Step 5: When coding injuries, be as specific as the documentation. Locate "Fall" in the index of the ICD-10-CM manual index and review ICD-10-CM code W19, remembering to use the seventh character, A, to indicate active treatment.

Example Encounter

An 88-year-old female patient with Medicare comes in for her yearly flu shot. After receiving a 0.5 mL single-shot dose of a preservative-free flu vaccine intramuscularly, the provider observes the patient for 15 minutes to monitor any adverse reactions.

CPT code: G0008

ICD-10-CM code: Z23

Step 1: Notice that the patient has Medicare insurance; therefore, she requires the use of an HCPCS code in place of a CPT intramuscular injection code.

Step 2: Locate "Administration" in the HCPCS manual index.

Step 3: Select "Influenza virus vaccine" and review HCPCS code G0008. Although the provider did spend an additional 15 minutes with the patient, the HCPCS manual instructs coding professionals to not bill an office visit procedure code if the reason for the encounter is only to administer a vaccination.

Step 4: Locate "Vaccination" in the ICD-10-CM index.

Step 5: Select "Encounter for" and review ICD-10-CM code Z23.

Example Encounter

A 67-year-old male patient has a confirmed case of lymphoma. He is placed under general anesthesia, and a flexible bronchoscope is inserted through the oral cavity to determine if the primary carcinoma has spread to the lung tissue. No lesions are observed in the bronchus. The bronchoscope is removed, and an incision is then made in the parasternal second left intercostal space, thus exposing the anterior mediastinal lymph nodes. Tissue samples from the lymph nodes are removed without complication. The incision is closed with sutures, and the patient is discharged.

CPT codes: 39010, 31622–51

ICD-10-CM code: C85.90

Step 1: Understand that two procedures are documented. The first is a bronchoscopy, meaning that a small tube with a camera is inserted through the nose or mouth to examine the airways and lungs. In this scenario, the procedure is for diagnostic purposes. The second procedure is a mediastinotomy, meaning that an incision is made into the parasternal intercostal space.

Step 2: Locate "Bronchoscopy" in the CPT manual index.

Step 3: Select "Diagnostic" and review CPT codes 31622–31624 and 31643.

Step 4: Locate "Mediastinotomy" in the CPT manual index.

Step 5: Select "Transthoracic approach" and review CPT code 39010.

Step 6: Locate and review the RVUs of both procedures and sequence appropriately. Modifier 51 should be appended to the procedure with the lowest RVU to indicate that multiple procedures were performed in the same session.

Step 7: Locate "Lymphoma" in the ICD-10-CM manual index and review ICD-10-CM code C85.90.

Example Encounter

A 60-year- heart old male patient is admitted to the intensive care unit with an acute chronic systolic failure exacerbation causing hypoxic respiratory failure. The patient is intubated, sedated, and started on 50 mg of ertapenem for a potential lung infection. Forty-five minutes was spent directly providing critical care for this patient.

CPT code: 99291

ICD-10-CM codes: I50.23, J96.91

Step 1: Understand that CPT guidelines define critical care as an illness or injury that acutely impairs one or more vital organ systems, where there is a high probability of imminent or life-threatening deterioration in the patient's condition. Additionally, the documentation should provide evidence of high-complexity MDM. In this scenario, the male patient has two life-threatening conditions, in which emergent intervention is provided to prevent further deterioration.

Step 2: Locate "Critical care services" in the CPT manual index.

Step 3: Select "Evaluation and management" and review CPT codes 99291–99292 and 99468–99476.

Step 4: Locate "Failure" in the ICD-10-CM manual index.

Step 5: Select "Heart," followed by "Systolic," followed by "Acute and chronic" and review ICD-10-CM codes I50.23.

Step 6: Locate "Failure" in the ICD-10-CM manual index.

Step 7: Select "Respiratory," followed by "With hypoxia" and review ICD-10-CM codes J96.91.

Example Encounter

A 55-year-old patient is admitted into the hospital for dialysis to treat end-stage renal disease. On day 13, the admitting physician spends 25 minutes discussing new management options for the patient's hypertension before sending a nurse to initiate the hemodialysis procedure.

CPT code: 99232

ICD-10-CM codes: I12.0, N18.6, Z99.2

Step 1: Understand that unless a physician is present for the entire duration of hemodialysis services, CPT guidelines advise physicians to only report the appropriate E/M code.

Step 2: Locate "Hospital services" in the CPT manual index.

Step 3: Select "Inpatient services," followed by "Subsequent hospital care" and review CPT codes 99231–99233.

Step 4: Locate "Disease" in the ICD-10-CM manual index.

Step 5: Select "Renal," followed by "End-stage" due to hypertension and review ICD-10-CM code I12.0. The additional notes provided advise using an additional code to identify the stage of CKD.

Step 6: Review ICD-10-CM codes N18.5 and N18.6. The additional notes provided advise using an additional code to identify dialysis status.

Step 7: Review ICD-10-CM code Z99.2.

Example Encounter

A 59-year-old male patient presents for a routine colonoscopy. During the procedure, a polyp is discovered.

CPT code: 45378

ICD-10-CM codes: Z12.11, K63.5

Step 1: Locate "Colonoscopy" in the CPT manual index.

Step 2: Select "Diagnostic" because the procedure is considered routine and not for purposes of treatment, and review CPT code 45378.

Step 3: Locate "Screening" in the ICD-10-CM manual index.

Step 4: Select "Colonoscopy" and review ICD-10-CM code Z12.11. The chapter notes provided on Z codes advise that if there is a finding during a screening, the finding may be used as an additional code.

Step 5: Locate "Polyp" in the ICD-10-CM manual index.

Step 6: Select "Colon" and review ICD-10-CM code K63.5.

Example Encounter

A patient with pre-existing hypertension presents to the office at 23 weeks of gestation for prenatal care. Her blood pressure is slightly elevated, and a transabdominal ultrasound shows that the fetus is small for dates. The provider advises the patient to rest and to follow up as normal. She is insured by a health plan that accepts the global obstetrical package.

CPT codes: 0502F, 76816

ICD-10-CM codes: O10.012, Z3A.23

Step 1: Notice that the patient is insured by a health plan that accepts the global obstetrical package. Instead of billing an E/M code, a placeholder code will be used instead.

Step 2: Locate "Pregnancy" in the CPT manual index.

Step 3: Select "Antepartum care" and review CPT codes 0500F–0502F.

Step 4: Locate "Ultrasound" in the CPT manual index.

Step 5: Select "Pregnant uterus" and review CPT codes 76801–76817, bearing in mind the gestational age of the fetus and the method that the images were obtained with.

Step 6: Locate "Pregnancy" in the ICD-10-CM manual index.

Step 7: Select complicating, followed by "Pregnancy," followed by "Essential," and review ICD-10-CM code O10.01-.

Step 8: Locate "Pregnancy" in the ICD-10-CM manual index.

Step 9: Select "Weeks of gestation" and locate the gestational age of the fetus.

Notice that the small-for-dates condition is not reported. The chapter notes contained in the ICD-10-CM manual explicitly state to only report fetal complications (O35. and O36.) when the fetal condition is responsible for modifying the care and management of the mother, which in this scenario, it is not.

EXAMPLE ENCOUNTER

A surgeon performs a posterior fusion on the L2–L5 of the spine on a 62-year-old patient due to degenerative disc disease.

CPT codes: 22612, 22614 × 2

ICD-10-CM code: M51.36

Step 1: Locate "Fusion" in the CPT manual index.

Step 2: Locate "Arthrodesis" in the CPT manual index.

Step 3: Understand that L signifies the lumbar spine in an orthopedic setting and that there are three lumbar fusion levels: L2-L3, L3-L4, and L4-L5. Select "Lumbar" and review CPT codes 22612, 22614, and 22630–22634. Notice that CPT code 22614 is an AOC and does not require a modifier.

Step 4: Locate "Degeneration" in the ICD-10-CM manual.

Step 5: Select "Intervertebral disc not elsewhere classifiable."

Step 6: Select "Lumbar region" and review ICD-10-CM code M51.36.

EXAMPLE ENCOUNTER

A selective catheter is placed into the thoracic aorta of an 81-year-old female patient with heart failure and a history of hypertension. The catheter is then manipulated into the left coronary artery and followed through into the right common carotid artery. Contrast injections are made, and digital imaging is performed. Upon completion, the catheter is removed, pressure is applied at the puncture site, and the patient is discharged.

CPT codes: 36215, 36216–59

ICD-10-CM code: I11.0

Step 1: Understand that the left coronary artery and the right common carotid artery are each considered to be their own vascular family. To determine the order of the arteries in the vascular family, locate Appendix O in the CPT manual.

Step 2: Locate "Catheterization" in the CPT manual index.

Step 3: Select "Aorta" and review CPT codes 36160–36215. Notice that contrast material and imaging is included in these procedures and is not reported as an additional charge. Additionally, modifier 59 is appended on CPT code 32616 to indicate that a different vascular family was evaluated in the same session.

Step 4: Locate "Failure" in the ICD-10-CM manual index.

Step 5: Select "Heart," followed by hypertension.

Step 6: Locate "Hypertension" in the ICD-10-CM manual index.

Step 7: Select "Heart," followed by "With heart failure," and review ICD-10-CM code I11.0.

Health Record Discrepancies

Occurrence of Health Record Discrepancy Before Patient Is Seen

Although the shift to electronic health records (EHRs) has provided multiple benefits — including better interpretation, faster delivery of test results, and improved coordination between healthcare professionals — medical record discrepancies remain a leading cause of death in the United States. For example, names, dates of birth, and social security numbers are commonly entered into a healthcare database incorrectly. This leads to duplicate medical records for the same patient, leaving one chart with outdated or irrelevant information. Additionally, due to the growing number of patient records, if a physician searches solely based on a patient's name or date of birth, he or she could select a chart for a completely different patient altogether. MDM based on incorrect or outdated medical records puts the patient's health at risk and a physician's licensure in jeopardy.

Reducing Registration Errors

Oftentimes, registration errors are the result of simple accidents. For example, ancillary staff may be pressured to obtain a patient's information within a certain time frame, leading to the entering or obtaining of misinformation. On the other hand, a high turnover rate may cause some to lack the knowledge needed to complete their assigned tasks correctly. One way an entity can work to counteract these errors is to **educate the registration staff** about how their actions have a direct impact on patient safety. Additionally, having a **clinical notification tool** available to identify possible duplicate charts can help deter the creation of multiple records. If having a clinical notification tool is not feasible, employees should ask patients if they have been to the hospital before. At least **three unique identifiers** in a patient's record should be confirmed prior to assuming the correct chart or creating a new one.

Chart Management Errors

Electronic templates were created as a guide to aid physicians with their documentation and validate that proper medical care was given. However, in some cases, templates are set to automatically populate certain data elements. Templates with this preset have resulted in inaccurate representations of patients' health and have also led to improper billing due to overdocumentation. Another chart management error may occur when a physician opts to "prestart" their notes prior to the patient encounter. If the patient is not seen, the note is usually deleted at a later time. However, other encounters have been inadvertently deleted instead, causing confusion between physicians and billing staff.

Reducing EHR Design Flaws

One of the best ways to reduce EHR design flaws is to educate physicians and other medical staff about the consequences of their actions. When individuals have an understanding that they are personally accountable and liable for what is entered into a medical record, errors are reduced because the time is now taken to review and verify the accuracy of what is documented. Additionally, practical steps can be taken to ensure that data elements essential to E/M leveling are not prepopulated and that copy-and-paste features are disabled.

Chart Completion Errors

Whether physicians are using an EHR or a paper chart to document a medical encounter, incomplete documentation errors remain a prevalent issue. One issue, for example, occurs when physicians have mistakenly opened and completed a chart note for an encounter that was either unsigned and/or incomplete for a different date of service. As a result, the integrity of that individual's medical chart is compromised and their health is put at risk during future encounters. Additionally, when a medical chart is incomplete, it makes it difficult — if not impossible — for a coding professional to accurately report the encounter, which could potentially put a physician or entity at risk for future audits, denials, and recoupments. It is necessary that physicians complete and sign their notes in a timely manner, usually within 48 hours of the encounter date, to avoid these repercussions.

Order and Data Entry Errors

Physicians are often able to issue a prescription through an EHR system. However, because prescription-based industries are rapidly advancing, newer medications may not yet be in the database. Although physicians and other clinical staff members generally have access to manually enter this information in the system, order entry errors occur when new medications are misspelled, resulting in erroneous entries and future prescription errors. Data entry errors can also occur due to spelling mistakes or typing errors when it comes to the entry of dates, quantities, vital signs, and other details. Physicians and clinical staff members should therefore take the time to ensure the correct entry of all information being entered into a medical chart.

Improving System Usability and Proper Use

Although improvements of the design and usability of EHR systems would help to eliminate the opportunity for error, physicians and other ancillary staff can take preventative steps now to improve system usability and ensure its proper use. For example, physicians and healthcare organizations can create and implement their own **policies and procedures handbook** that relates directly to the appropriate use of an EHR system. Topics such as copy and paste and template use should be addressed. Additionally, **adequate training** on EHR systems and their appropriate use should be prearranged upon employment and assessed on an annual basis thereafter. Lastly, an **internal reporting system** can also be created to identify, report, and correct EHRs and/or EHR-related issues promptly.

Provider Queries

Compliance

Query

A query is a tool used to **communicate** with a physician or other qualified healthcare practitioners to **clarify** documentation in a medical record and to ensure accurate procedural and diagnosis coding. For example, a query could be used to **resolve** conflicting documentation, to determine if a condition documented in the history section of the medical record is active and unresolved and/or to seek clarification if a documented diagnosis does not appear to be clinically supported. Additionally, a query is not used to rectify every discrepancy seen in the medical record, nor is it used to increase reimbursement.

When to Not Send a Query

Although the ability to query a physician is a useful tool to clarify documentation and ensure coding accuracy, all appropriate steps should be taken by the coding professional to resolve the issue on their own first, perhaps by consulting facility-specific coding guidelines. Additionally, it is the responsibility of the coder to know and understand the anatomy of the body system they are assigned to code. A physician should not be queried regarding a coder's knowledge deficit. For example, if a physician documents that the cecum colon from the appendix to the ascending part of the colon was removed, that would involve the entire body part. Therefore, there would be no need to query the physician to find out if the procedure involved a partial or total removal.

Multiple-Choice Queries

A multiple-choice query is formulated based on clinical indicators in the medical record. A multiple-choice query allows the physician or other qualified healthcare practitioners to choose one or more listed diagnoses and/or other related documentation resolutions. The query should be written in a nonleading format, meaning that the qualified healthcare practitioner should not feel pressured or encouraged to choose one or more choices over another. As an example, if a provider documents that the occurrence of diabetes occurred at age 10, a multiple-choice query may be sent to the provider inquiring if the diabetes can be further specified as type 1 or type 2 based on the documented history of the patient.

Yes-or-No Queries

A yes-or-no query is formulated based on clinical indicators in the medical record and should be written in a manner that allows the physician or other qualified healthcare practitioner to respond with a "yes" or a "no." Yes-or-no queries can be used to substantiate a diagnosis found in imaging or pathology, clarify conflicts in documentation, and to confirm causal relationships when the documentation lends itself to it. As an example, a medical record contains a current diagnosis of sepsis with no documented cause; however, a urinary tract infection (UTI) is noted in the medical history. In this instance because an untreated UTI is known to cause sepsis, an appropriate yes-or-no query to the provider may be, "Is the sepsis due to or the result of the recent UTI? Please document yes or no."

Open-Ended Queries

An open-ended query is formulated based on clinical indicators in the medical record and should be written in a manner that allows the provider to express themselves freely. This type of query is commonly used to clarify or substantiate a diagnosis based on documented results. As an example, a medical record notes that a patient is admitted due to difficulty breathing, but he also presents with a fever and a cough that produces yellow mucus. A sputum culture was collected and tested positive for bacteria; however, the provider fails to provide a definitive diagnosis. In this instance, an open-ended query to the provider may be, "Based on your clinical judgment, please provide a diagnosis that could encompass the following conditions: difficulty breathing, a temperature of 101°F, and a positive culture for *Klebsiella pneumoniae*."

Noncompliant Query

A noncompliant query is one that encourages or leads a provider or other healthcare practitioner to a specific conclusion, clarification, disease, or illness. A query would also be considered noncompliant if it failed to have the supporting clinical indicators in the medical record. Additionally, a query should never include information on reimbursement and/or question the provider's clinical judgment. When creating a query, ask yourself: Could this query be debated or challenged as noncompliant? If you are unsure or if the answer is yes, consider changing the query. If a noncompliant query is found, inform a supervisor, manager, and/or compliance officer immediately.

Example

Clinical scenario: A male patient with prostate cancer is seen for the first time by an oncologist. The oncologist documents a problem-focused history, a detailed exam, and decision making of moderate complexity.

Query: Based on the problem-focused history intake, only a 99201 E/M code may be billed. However, the rest of your note qualifies for a 99203 E/M code. Would you like to review your history intake?

Rationale: This type of query is inappropriate because it specifically relates to reimbursement. A more compliant course of action could be to recommend that the provider be educated on documentation improvement techniques.

Documenting Queries

There are several types of queries, which include open-ended, multiple-choice, yes-or-no, and verbal queries. All queries, regardless of format, should be **concise** and **factual** in terms of clinical indicators, should include the reason that clarification is needed, and should be **nonleading** — meaning that the qualified healthcare practitioner should not feel pressured or encouraged to choose or answer in a certain way. Additionally, a query should never include information on reimbursement. Any query or change made by the practitioner to the medical record should be considered permanent and should be retained for compliance and/or auditing. When unsure of whether to query or the documentation guidelines of a query, reach out to your compliance officer or request a copy of the organization's query policy.

Compliance of Queries

A noncompliant query is subject to serious consequences. Leading a provider or other healthcare professional to a diagnosis or involving reimbursement in a query, especially when done as a pattern, can lead to target audits, monetary recoupments, or fraudulent prosecution. A target audit involves an internal and/or external review of a procedure, provider, or coder aimed at identifying errors. This type of review can be time-consuming and can result in delayed payments or a retraction of previously administered funds, commonly known as a monetary recoupment. Although not common, a consequence of a noncompliant query may involve fraudulent prosecution because it has the appearance of impropriety and does not meet the high standard of ethics required of a healthcare entity.

AHIMA Code of Ethics and Physician Queries

The American Health Information Management Association (AHIMA) code of ethics has been established to offer guidance and principles in the decision-making process of documentation and billing. The AHIMA code of ethics encourages clinical documentation improvement and provides examples of behaviors and situations that assist in simplifying how to interpret the ethical standards they set. To avoid the appearance of impropriety and to incorporate best practices into the healthcare industry, AHIMA has developed ethical standards related to queries that include the following: Create and review query policies annually, queries must only reflect facts pertaining to the required clarification, queries must obtain clinical indicators that are related to the episode of care, and queries should be retained and considered as a permanent part of the health record.

Verbal Queries

A verbal query is formulated based on clinical indicators in the medical record and allows the provider or other healthcare practitioner to express themselves over the phone or in person. A verbal query may be asked in a manner that elicits an open-ended response or a yes-or-no response. Multiple-choice options may also be verbalized to the healthcare practitioner in a manner that allows them to choose which action or diagnosis would successfully resolve a discrepancy within the medical record. Also note that, when a query has been asked and answered verbally, it must still be documented in the medical record with a note of what clarification was needed, why clarification was needed, the clinical indicators involved, the options the healthcare practitioner was presented with (if any), the outcome, and the exact date and time that the query occurred, followed by the provider's signature to indicate agreement.

Query Opportunities

Example of Compliant Multiple-Choice Query

Physician documentation: A 30-year-old established female patient was seen for her annual gynecological visit. A bilateral breast exam was performed with a lump noted on the upper inner quadrant of the right breast. A Pap smear was collected with sexually transmitted disease cultures. The patient was counseled on performing self-breast exams monthly, a referral was provided for a mammogram, and counseling was given on safe-sex practices.

Query: Did the annual exam that you performed result in normal findings or abnormal findings? Please select one.

Reasoning: In this scenario, knowing whether or not the gynecological exam performed resulted in normal or abnormal findings is essential to choosing a correct diagnosis code. This type of multiple-choice query does not pressure the physician to choose one option over the other, and both options are clinically reasonable and valid.

Example of Noncompliant Multiple-Choice Query

Physician documentation: A 45-year-old male patient was admitted 2 days ago due to a gastrointestinal bleed, which has since resolved. His hemoglobin levels dropped to 8 g/dL, and one unit of blood was transfused. Patient is being discharged and advised to take 45 mg of iron per day over the next week.

Query: Can you please specify whether the patient has anemia, acute posthemorrhagic anemia, or iron-deficiency anemia secondary to blood loss?

Reasoning: Because anemia is not an established diagnosis in the physician's documentation, it should not be mentioned in the query. In this scenario, an open-ended query should be used to establish a diagnosis.

Example of Compliant Yes-or-No Query

Physician documentation: An 88-year-old male patient is seen in the ED with complaints of pain and bleeding on his lower back. The patient reports little to no physical activity throughout the day because he gets tired easily. A physical exam reveals a deep-tissue ulcer on the coccyx. The patient is admitted and given antibiotics intravenously.

Query: Is the ulcer due to constant pressure on the skin? Please document yes or no.

Reasoning: In order to select the most specific and accurate diagnosis, further specification is needed to determine the type of ulcer that the patient has. Because the physician documented "little to no physical activity" and bedsores are the leading cause of ulcers in elderly people, the query is clinically relevant.

Example of Noncompliant Yes-or-No Query

Clinical Scenario: A 27-year-old established female patient was seen by her gynecologist with complaints of missed periods for the past 6 months. The history portion of the medical record reveals multiple follicular cysts, and a physical exam shows hirsutism. A recent lab reports elevated testosterone levels exceeding 60 ng/dL.

Query: Please document if you agree that the patient has polycystic ovarian syndrome.

Rationale: This type of yes-or-no query leads the provider to a specific illness that is not already mentioned in the medical report. In this scenario, an open-ended query would be more appropriate.

Example of Compliant Open-Ended Query

Physician documentation: A 72-year-old female patient is seen in the ED with complaints of difficulty breathing and general body aches. A physical exam reveals that the patient has a fever, chest congestion, and altered mental status. A sputum culture is collected and tests positive for bacteria. The patient is started on intravenous fluids and oxygen.

Query: Based on your clinical judgment, please provide a diagnosis that would encompass a positive bacteria culture, chest congestion, and fever.

Reasoning: In this scenario, clinical indicators are brought to the provider in order to substantiate a diagnosis that is currently not present in the documentation.

Example of Noncompliant Open-Ended Query

Physician documentation: A 61-year-old established patient with a history of smoking is seen today complaining of a cough and difficulty breathing. Bilateral breath sounds reveal fluid in the lungs. A culture is collected and is positive for bacteria. I have prescribed vancomycin and advised the patient to follow up in 3 days.

Query: Can you please specify the type of pneumonia you are treating?

Reasoning: This query is rather unclear for a physician who is not aware of coding conventions. Although the query is aimed at determining which bacteria caused the pneumonia, a physician may simply respond with a general statement, such as "severe" or "bacterial." In this scenario, a multiple-choice query would ensure the needed response.

Example of Compliant Verbal Query

Physician documentation: A 56-year-old female patient experiencing swollen lymph nodes is seen for a follow-up visit to discuss the results of her open axillary biopsy that occurred last week. The patient is given multiple treatment options, including the success rates, risks, and side effects. She opts to begin radiation treatment next week.

Query: Because the documentation is not specific, I spoke with the physician today regarding the biopsy results in the patient's chart, which are positive for diffuse large-cell lymphoma, and asked whether or not he agreed with this. The physician confirmed that the counsel he gave to the patient was surrounding this diagnosis.

Reasoning: Although just a short statement, the documentation explains why a query was needed, the clinical indicators for such a query, when the discussion with the physician took place, and what the agreed-upon outcome was.

Example of Noncompliant Verbal Query

Physician documentation: A 14-year-old new patient was seen with complaints of sharp pain and bruising on the upper portion of the right leg. The patient's mother reports that the patient fell down the stairs while running. Imaging results show the proximal end of the right femur with positioning similar to that seen today in the office. The patient was referred to the orthopedic surgeon for follow-up care.

Query: The physician agreed that the patient has an intertrochanteric fracture of the proximal right femur.

Reasoning: Verbal queries should contain the actual question that was raised to the physician and give the essence of what was discussed with the provider. The current query insinuates that the discussion was leading and was not based on clinical indicators found in the note.

Regulatory Compliance

Integrity of Health Records

Documentation Cloning

Documentation cloning, also referred to as copying and pasting, is when the documentation for one encounter appears **identical** or **similar** to the documentation from another encounter. Although this is typically seen in electronic medical records due to features such as copy and paste, autofill, and pulling information forward from a previous encounter, it can also be seen in handwritten charts. Although these methods of documenting are not prohibited and may be used at times when it relates to the patient's history or ROS, the same patient should not have the same exact complaint, symptoms, physical examination, and/or treatment on **each** encounter and their documentation certainly should not resemble that of a different patient's encounter.

Dangers Surrounding Cloned Documentation

Documentation cloning has the potential to lead to errors in patient care. It has been reported that information has at times been cloned into the **incorrect chart**. Another danger includes **contradictions** within the medical record. For example, if a provider copies a negative complete ROS from a previous encounter, but the patient presents with abdominal pain, there is now a discrepancy that will need to be clarified and amended. Additionally, CMS has deemed the billing of cloned documentation as a **misrepresentation** of services because it is unclear what previous history was reviewed and what new information was collected. Consider, too, that if the documentation is the same as or similar to a previous encounter, it **lacks** the **medical necessity** to support why the patient was seen again.

Fraud

Fraud occurs when a provider deliberately bills for a service that was never provided and/or reports a service with a higher reimbursement rate than the service that was actually provided. For example, a dermatologist in Florida falsely diagnosed multiple elderly patients with skin cancer and surgically removed the "malignant" portion of skin in an effort to obtain greater revenue from Medicare. This type of intentional behavior is not only illegal, but it is also unethical. If a person is found to be involved in fraudulent activity, those persons are subject to monetary penalties and/or incarceration. If you become aware of fraudulent activity, a complaint can be filed online with the Office of Inspector General (OIG) at www.oig.hhs.gov/.

Abuse

Abuse occurs when a service reported is misused, not medically necessary, or overcharged. For example, a physician documents that a mass located on a patient's leg took 30 minutes to excise but fails to document the reason for the excessive amount of time. If the physician were to report the procedure with modifier 22, indicating increased procedural services, this would be considered abuse because the medical necessity to substantiate such a reimbursement is lacking. Whether the intent is deliberate or not, abuse is considered illegal and if persons are found to be involved, they are subject to monetary penalties and/or incarceration. The best way to avoid this improper billing practice is to participate in self-audits and to be fully aware of the compliance programs created by an organization or entity by which you are employed.

WASTE

Waste occurs when a service is overused, resulting in unnecessary cost to Medicare and Medicaid. Usually, there is no knowledge or malicious intent behind these rendered services. For example, a low-risk obstetric patient is told to come in for weekly ultrasounds in her first trimester. Because the patient is not at risk and most fetal organs are either not developed and/or cannot be visualized in the first trimester, this is considered an unnecessary cost. If found to be involved in waste, those persons are subject to monetary penalties, which can include the repayment of services found to be wasteful. The best way to avoid this improper billing practice is to participate in self-audits and be fully aware of the compliance programs created by an organization or entity by which you are employed.

ADDENDUM TO MEDICAL RECORD

An addendum is a correction, deletion, or amendment to a completed medical record. If the addendum occurs in an EHR, the system must be configured to allow for such changes. An EHR should also be capable of tracking who made the changes, the reason for the changes, and the date and time of such changes, as well as the original entry. If any of these listed elements is not included in an EHR's functionality, it should be manually entered. On the other hand, if the medical record is handwritten, the correction should be made with a single black permanent line. It should be noted that when an alteration is made *after* submission to an insurance carrier, the alteration is considered a deliberate misrepresentation of facts.

PATIENT IDENTIFIERS

Patient identifiers are required by the Health Insurance Portability and Accountability Act (HIPAA) in order to maintain and protect a person's private health information (PHI). Patient identifiers not only help to maintain a patient's privacy and security, but they also minimize the risk of a healthcare provider and/or other ancillary staff from unknowingly adding incorrect health information or divulging results that were thought to belong to a different patient. A patient identifier may include, but is not limited to, special alerts when accessing an EHR, a medical identification number, and/or confirmation of the date of birth and full name of the patient.

AUDITS AND AUDIT TRAILS

An audit is an internal or external **review** performed to compare medical documentation against what was actually reported to ensure proper coding and compliance with policies and procedures. Additionally, some electronic health systems maintain an audit trail, which captures the information of a user who accesses a medical record; when and where they accessed it from; and what, if any, documentation was added, amended, or deleted. This information can also be used to identify trends in how health records are being used. Audits and audit trails ensure the integrity of a medical record by **creating legal liability** to maintain accurate documentation and confidentiality.

SIGNATURE REQUIREMENTS

Regardless of the authorship of a medical entry, it must be authenticated with a handwritten or electronic signature or attestation. This type of authentication **identifies** each individual's contribution to the medical record and **validates** the services and/or procedures that were provided. In general, a medical entry should be signed or attested to within 24 to 72 hours of when the service was provided, with some exceptions that are dependent on pathology results, transcriptionist delays, etc. Before reporting any codes to an insurance carrier, be sure that the medical entry is authenticated with the appropriate signature requirements because not doing so will risk denials and potential audits.

Appropriate and Inappropriate Provider Attestations

An attestation is a statement from a physician that validates his/her review and participation in the care rendered to a patient. Oftentimes, teaching physicians will document attestations when a patient is seen by a medical student, resident, or fellow, in order to confirm their presence and/or participation in key portions of the treatment. For example, if a resident has written a medical entry and the provider personally performed the key components required to bill an E/M code, an **appropriate** attestation may be, "I saw and evaluated the patient. I reviewed the resident's note and agree with the findings and plan as documented." An **inappropriate** attestation for the same situation may be, "I discussed the case with the resident and I agree" or "The patient was seen and evaluated." Both examples lack the specificity required to prove that the provider was actually present during the treatment or participated in the patient's care.

Role of OIG in Medical Records

The Office of Inspector General (OIG) is an independent, government-run agency with a mission to detect and combat waste, fraud, and abuse in the medical system, specifically within Medicare and Medicaid. Each year, the OIG creates various projects known as work plans, in order to assess potential oversights and risks within the healthcare field. For example, in 2012, a work plan was created to focus on fraud vulnerabilities related to EHRs. Their investigation concluded that some organizations were not able to determine whether a provider had copied and pasted medical record entries and advised CMS to encourage the use of provider audit logs. The OIG's workplans can be accessed by visiting https://oig.hhs.gov/reports-and-publications/workplan/active-item-table.asp. A regular review of this information allows coding professionals and physicians to fix their own unintended errors before becoming the target of an audit.

Effective Compliance Plan

A healthcare compliance plan consists of written policies and procedures to ensure that physicians and nonclinical staff observe the regulations and laws that relate to healthcare practices. An effective healthcare compliance plan should include the following elements, as outlined by the OIG. First, each healthcare practice should have a **designated compliance officer** that others can reach out to when they discover or suspect a potential violation. Second, there should be consistent and appropriate training and education regarding HIPAA and the EHR systems that are used. A third aspect of an effective compliance program includes conducting internal monitoring and auditing of all reported charges. Finally, a compliance plan should outline the standards of the practice and the disciplinary and corrective action that will be taken if those standards are violated.

Payer-Specific Guidelines

Coding Rejections and Denials

A **rejection** is a claim for medical services and/or supplies that cannot be submitted and/or processed, usually due to incorrect patient information. Once a rejected claim is corrected and resubmitted, it may then be reviewed for payment. A **denial** is a claim for medical services and/or supplies that has been received and processed by Medicare, Medicaid, a commercial insurance carrier, or third-party payer, but it is deemed to be unpayable for one or more reasons. An explanation of benefits statement linked to the claim provides a physician or entity with detailed reasons for the denial, providing them with an opportunity to correct the claim and resubmit it for payment.

Common Causes of Coding Denials

One common cause of coding denials includes **code changes**. Each fiscal year, updates are made to the ICD-10-CM, CPT, and HCPC Level II manuals. If a coder does not personally review these updates or if an entity does not update its EHR system, an outdated code may be selected. A second cause of denials is **varying payer guidelines**. For example, some private insurance carriers will not pay for any service related to birth-control or abortion, due to their associated religious background. Other denial reasons include:

- incorrect modifier use
- submitting claims 90 days or more after services were rendered
- a lack of medical necessity.

Prevention Strategies to Reduce Coding Denials

Understanding the cause of most coding denials can help a coding professional work on a proactive solution to prevent them. For example, if a coder knows that incorrect modifier use can lead to a coding denial, they can familiarize themselves with how to use the code edits provided by CMS. Another crucial element to avoid common mistakes that lead to denials is to participate in ongoing **training and education**. These sessions are useful resources to stay up to date with any coding and/or payer changes. Additionally, some entities have built a dedicated **edits and denials team** whose sole focus is to research, appeal, and resubmit claims that have previously been denied. Because of their experience and knowledge, most entities experience greater productivity and revenue with their claim submissions.

MPPR Rule

When multiple procedures are performed on the same day and by the same physician or by multiple physicians in the same practice, the reimbursement of such procedures may be subject to the **multiple procedure payment reduction (MPPR)** rule. Under the MPPR rule, typically the primary procedure will be reimbursed at 100% of the allowable amount, although all secondary procedures will be paid at a lesser value, usually 50% or 25% of the allowable amount. This is because most of the procedures in the CPT manual include both pre- and post-procedure work, thus causing an overlap. The MPPR rule was originally designed by CMS for patients insured by Medicare and Medicaid; however, other insurance carriers have adopted the same or similar MPPR concepts.

Exceptions

Not all procedure codes in the CPT manual are subject to the MPPR rule. One exception involves E/M codes that are reported with **modifier 25**, indicating that a separately identifiable service was rendered on the same day. Additionally, **add-on procedures** and **procedures exempt from modifier 51**, as so stated in the CPT manual, are also excluded from the reimbursement reduction. The assigned value for these CPT codes was given on the notion that they would be reported with other procedures. Therefore, an additional reimbursement reduction would not be necessary or fair. For a full list of add-on and modifier 51-exempt CPT codes, see Appendix F of the CPT manual.

Medicare, Medicaid, and Private Health Insurance

Medicare is a federal system of health insurance for individuals past the age of 65 and for those under the age of 65 with disabilities or end-stage renal disease. **Medicaid** is also a federal system of health insurance, but it is monitored and administered by each state. Medicaid serves as a free or low-cost source of health coverage for individuals who are considered to have a low income, children, pregnant women, elderly adults, and those with disabilities. Because Medicare and Medicaid are public health systems, the coverage an individual receives from them and the providers with whom they are treated by can be quite limited. **Private health insurance** is coverage offered by an insurance company or broker. Individuals who elect to have private health insurance have the ability to reduce or increase its cost by customizing a plan to fit their needs.

Medicare Coverage

Medicare offers several coverage options to its enrollees. Medicare **Part A** covers inpatient hospital stays and care received in a skilled nursing facility, hospice program, or home health care. **Part B** covers services and preventative care rendered by a physician, outpatient care, and medical supplies. **Part C**, otherwise known as a Medicare Advantage plan, bundles Part A and Part B into one plan dispensed by a private insurance carrier contracted with Medicare. Add-on coverage is also available, such as **Part D** for prescription drugs, or **Medigap** to help offset out-of-pocket expenses.

Payer-Specific Guidelines When Reporting Anesthesia Services

When it comes to reporting the time for anesthesia services, the CPT manual advises that the start time begins when the anesthesiologist begins preparing the patient for induction and ends when the patient is safely placed under postoperative supervision. However, it also adds that the time "*may be reported as is customary in the local area.*" For example, Horizon Blue Cross and Blue Shield allows physicians to round their time to the closest 15-minute interval, whereas Medicare requires exact time reporting. Other variations may occur with some states that recognize anesthesia assistants and others that do not.

Payer-Specific Guidelines When Reporting Preventative Services

Because payer-specific guidelines differ, a coding professional will need to familiarize themselves with what is required of them when reporting. When it comes to preventative services, Medicare requires that certain specialties bill an HCPCS Level II code, whereas many private health insurance carriers only accept CPT codes. For example, when reporting a gynecological preventative visit for an established 60-year-old female patient who is covered under Medicare, HCPCS Level II code G0101 should be reported instead of CPT code 99396 to avoid receiving a claim denial and vice versa.

Creating Facility-Specific Guidelines

Facility-specific guidelines are useful tools that promote consistent and accurate code assignment within a coding department. They also serve to help educate new hires on what is required from the insurance carriers to which they report and the laws that govern the state. Facility-specific guidelines also serve as a helpful resource when appealing claim denials because they may contain the official guidelines from the ICD-10-CM, CPT, and HCPCS manuals, journals published by AHIMA, as well as documents published by the Centers for Disease Control and Prevention, CMS, the American Hospital Association, and the AMA.

Patient Safety Indicators (PSIs) and Hospital-Acquired Conditions (HACs)

PSIs

Patient safety indicators (PSIs) are 27 quality measures that were developed by the Agency for Healthcare Research and Quality (AHRQ) in 2002 as a way to identify potential safety issues within an inpatient hospital setting. These potential safety issues include hospital complications or adverse events that follow a procedure and/or childbirth. PSIs are generated using discharge data derived from administrative databases. Once obtained, PSIs can and have been used to generate respective hospital rankings in terms of safety within the United States.

Contributions of Coding Professionals to PSIs

PSIs are generated using discharge data derived from administrative databases, which include diagnosis and procedures codes, admission information, and patient demographics. A coding professional can improve an entity's PSIs by accurately representing an admission through their coding. Doing so ensures confidence that the PSIs reflect the correct care and outcomes. Additionally, a coding professional serves as the first line of defense to identify problems related to hospital complications and/or adverse events, which in turn leads to prompt prevention strategies. On the other hand, improper coding can negatively impact an entity's PSIs. Although most coding professionals are trained in terminology and documentation guidelines, many clinicians are not. This can lead to an inaccurate clinical picture if the diagnosis codes are assigned without consideration of disease progression or clinical context.

PSI 90: Patient Safety for Selected Indicators

PSI 90 is a combined measure of multiple indicators that reflect a marker of general patient safety during the administration of inpatient care. These indicators include the observed versus expected ratios of pressure ulcers, postoperative respiratory failure and sepsis, and in-hospital falls that result in hip fractures, as well as multiple other components. Because PSI 90 is represented by a single metric, it can easily be used to either review a hospital's performance over time or to compare its measurement against the national, regional, state, and/or provider average. CMS will commonly use PSI 90 as a way to assess performance and evaluate facility reimbursement.

Improving Hospital's Performance Rating in Relation to PSI 06: Iatrogenic Pneumothorax

An iatrogenic pneumothorax is an adverse event from a medical procedure that causes an individual's lung to collapse; it is considered a serious, life-threatening condition. AHRQ provides preventative measures that hospitals and professional coders can take to ensure patient safety and quality coding. For example, in order to reduce injury, AHRQ recommends the use of bedside ultrasound guidance during a catheter placement. When coding, be aware that pneumothorax should not be reported when the condition is suspected and/or being ruled out. Rather, code only confirmed conditions established by means of a chest X-ray or CT scan.

Improving Hospital's Performance Rating in Relation to PSI 12: Postoperative Deep Vein Thrombosis (DVT) and Pulmonary Embolism

A deep vein thrombosis (DVT) is a blood clot that forms in the deep veins of the body, sometimes causing pain or swelling. If not treated promptly, part of the clot can travel into the lungs, causing a blockage known as a pulmonary embolism. As of 2019, pulmonary emboli were considered the most common, but preventable, causes of death among hospitalized patients. When it comes to DVTs, AHRQ urges physicians to consider starting mechanical and/or pharmacologic prophylaxis on day 0, even without symptoms, if the patient is at intermediate risk of developing a DVT. Coding professionals are encouraged to educate themselves and providers on DVT guidelines and order sets in the EHR.

Effects of PSIs on Revenue

In 2003, CMS established a pay-for-performance initiative. The pay-for-performance initiative was designed to provide an incentive to hospitals to hold physicians accountable for their actions, enhance the quality of care, and to improve patient outcomes. Through this initiative, if a physician can provide evidence of compliance and improvement through PSIs, they will be rewarded with higher reimbursement rates for the services they render. On the other hand, hospitals that show little to no improvement in PSIs could face monetary penalties. It is important to note that since its establishment, other private healthcare payers have also instituted their own versions of pay-for-performance systems.

HACs

Hospital-acquired conditions (HACs), also known as nosocomial infections, are illnesses that arise 48–72 hours after an individual is admitted for inpatient hospital or facility stay. These illnesses arise due to errors, injuries, and/or infections that could have been prevented by the healthcare staff. Common HACs include central line-associated bloodstream infections, catheter-associated UTIs, pneumonias resulting from growing bacteria in ventilators, postoperative fungal infections, hip fractures due to falls, pressure sores, objects left in a patient during surgery, and accidental lacerations. The longer a patient remains in an inpatient hospital or facility, the higher the likelihood of developing an HAC.

HAC Reduction Program

The HAC Reduction Program was established in 2014 by CMS to encourage general acute-care hospitals "to improve patients' safety and reduce the number of conditions that people experience from their time in a hospital." Under this program, hospitals are ranked against each other on a scale of 1 to 10. Where they stand is based on the number of complications that resulted from being in a hospital. Medicare and Medicaid penalize the worst 25 percent by reducing reimbursement on medical claims by 1 percent in the following fiscal year. Although it may not sound like much, this reduction often amounts to millions of dollars each year.

Reducing and Eliminating HACs

The Centers for Disease Control and Prevention has provided prevention strategies aimed at detecting, preventing, and reducing HACs in the healthcare field. Included in their suggestions are that hospitals have a competency-based training program for hand hygiene that is performed upon hire and then repeated annually. Personnel are also encouraged to wear personal protective equipment (PPE) when interacting with patients who may be at a higher risk for developing an infection. Additionally, training should be provided on an annual basis regarding the appropriate use of medical supplies, such as the insertion of urinary catheters, the proper fit and function of respiratory devices, and the correct technique for the insertion of central venous catheters.

Impact of Coding Professionals on HACs

Because of the impact that HACs and PSIs have on a hospital, a coding professional must ensure that their work is accurate and is based on the information collected from the entire medical record. To report any information incorrectly could have a negative impact on a hospital's revenue cycle and reputation. Additionally, the accurate reporting and capturing of HACs and PSIs by coding professionals allows hospitals to review the quality of care that they are providing and implement practices to create a safer healthcare environment for their patients.

Example of Deciding to Report or Not Report an HAC

A coding professional may look at a medical record and find that a urinary tract infection (UTI) is documented. Because UTI is a common HAC, it could be considered appropriate for the coder to assume that the infection occurred after the patient was admitted and was therefore preventable. If that were actually the case, a coder could report the UTI with POA indicator N and payment would be denied correctly. However, a closer look into the entire chart reveals that, although the patient was admitted for a concurring condition, there were also documented complaints of pelvic pain and dysuria. In that case, because the symptoms were present, the infection would be considered POA and the indicator associated with it would be Y, which means that CMS would pay for the treatment.

HIPAA Guidelines

HIPAA and HIPAA Privacy Rule

The Health Insurance Portability and Accountability Act (HIPAA), is a **federal law** established in 1996 to **protect** a patient's private health information (PHI) and electronic protected health information (ePHI) from being disclosed without a patient's written consent. PHI and ePHI include past, present, or future health conditions, treatment, payments, and demographics. Falling under the umbrella of HIPAA is a subcategory of **national standards**, known as the HIPAA Privacy Rule. The HIPAA Privacy Rule was designed to ensure the **safety** of personal health information that is transmitted or received electronically. HIPAA and the HIPAA Privacy Rule are in place to reduce the level of risk associated with a potential violation and/or breach and to promote high-quality health care.

Compliance with HIPAA Privacy Rule

The HIPAA Privacy Rule mandates that all covered entities follow the national standards that it sets forth. A covered entity is any person(s) or organization that provides treatment or payment in the healthcare field. This includes every **healthcare provider** who transmits health information electronically for the purpose of obtaining eligibility, authorizations, and payment. It also includes **healthcare clearinghouses** that process ePHI from one entity to another. **Business associates**, such as a third-party billing or consulting agency, also fall under the category of a covered entity if their function involves the use of PHI and ePHI. Finally, any individual or group **health plans**, including dental, vision, health maintenance organizations, and employer-sponsored or church-sponsored health plans, are also covered entities if they are providing or paying for the cost of medical care.

Disclosure of PHI Without Authorization

Under the HIPAA Privacy Rule, a covered entity may disclose PHI without an individual's authorization in some circumstances. These include disclosing PHI or ePHI for the purpose of treatment and payment. For example, a physician may submit PHI directly to a patient's health plan without the patient's permission. A covered entity may also release PHI or ePHI to a government agency if they have confirmed exposure to a communicable disease and notification is required by law. When a patient is underage and confirmed to be a victim of abuse, neglect, or domestic violence, a covered entity may disclose PHI or ePHI to the appropriate authorities. Additional permitted disclosures may be given at the request of the individual, for healthcare operations, for the opportunity to agree or object, for incidental use, or for research and/or public health purposes when the patient identifiers have been removed.

Steps to Ensure Compliance with HIPAA and HIPAA Privacy Rule

To ensure compliance with HIPAA and the HIPAA Privacy Rule, covered entities should implement three types of safeguards to protect patient information from disclosure to any unauthorized person(s). The first type of safeguard is a technical safeguard. For example, HIPAA requires ePHI to be **encrypted** so that if there is a breach, all ePHI is unreadable and undecipherable. A covered entity should also implement physical safeguards, such as a **HIPAA Policies and Procedures** handbook, which governs the entry and restrictions of accessing ePHI and PHI. The final safeguard is administrative, and it includes conducting **risk assessments** to identify which ePHI is being used and where a potential breach could occur. Covered entities are also required to develop a **contingency plan**, which would ensure access and protection of ePHI in case of an emergency.

Ways Policy and Procedure Documents Can Deter an Entity from Complying with HIPAA

If a policy and procedure document is **too long** or **too complex**, an entity may be deterred from either creating such a document or understanding and complying with it. Instead, policy and procedure documents should be concise, logical, and easy to understand. Although it may be challenging to create a concise document that addresses PHI, ePHI, and HIPAA, AHIMA encourages policy and procedure documents to be no longer than four pages. Additionally, some entities have made their policy and procedure documents accessible online via shared folders. Not only does this allow more flexibility to update, maintain, or make changes, but it also encourages usability and convenience to its users.

HIPAA Violations

A **HIPAA violation** is when a covered entity fails to comply with any of its regulations. A HIPAA violation can be considered deliberate or unintentional. However, regardless of how it is perceived, a covered entity will be held responsible for the damages, which may include employee dismissal, fines ranging from $100 to $50,000 per violation, civil penalties, prison sentences up to 10 years, or a combination of these. Although at times the Office of Civil Rights has used their discretion to waive civil penalties for unintentional HIPAA violations, unfamiliarity with the HIPAA regulations is not an excuse. All medical personnel should be educated and take appropriate steps to ensure compliance.

Breach

A **breach** is the disclosure of PHI and/or ePHI outside of those allowed by the HIPAA Privacy Rule. HIPAA requires a breach to be reported within 60 days of its discovery to the affected individuals by First-Class Mail or by email. A covered entity is also required to notify the Secretary of Health & Human Services (HHS) of a breach. If a breach involves fewer than 500 individuals, notification may be delayed up to 60 days following the end of the calendar year in which the breach was discovered. If a breach involves more than 500 individuals, a covered entity is required to notify the secretary of HHS within 60 days of discovering the breach. This can be done by visiting the HHS website and submitting a "Notice of Breach" form. In some cases, a breach affecting more than 500 residents located in the same state may require media notification through a press release within 60 days of discovering a breach.

Risks Associated with ePHI

Although computers, phones, and tablets provide a fast and efficient way to document, communicate, and send information, risks are involved if their use is not monitored for privacy and security. Such risks include, but are not limited to, **theft or loss** of a device, **improper disposal** of a device, or **interception** of a transmission by an unauthorized person. For example, although it is okay to send ePHI with a mobile device, if it is sent in a text message to another mobile device that is turned off, the message can temporarily be routed through the Internet or a cellular network of telecommunications providers, resulting in a breach. Additionally, under the HIPAA Privacy Rule, a patient has the right to access and amend their medical record. If text messages are used to communicate ePHI, they are subject to this. However, failing to provide access and the ability to amend such messages would be considered a **violation** of the HIPAA Privacy Rule.

Ensuring Compliance with HIPAA and HIPAA Privacy Rule

To ensure compliance with HIPAA and the HIPAA Privacy Rule, coding professionals should implement safe habits to protect patient information from disclosure to any unauthorized person(s). For example, when creating new login credentials, choose a strong password that includes a variety of letters, numbers, and symbols. A coding professional should only access information that is necessary to perform their basic job responsibilities. PHI should never be discarded in a trash receptacle; rather, it should be destroyed or shredded immediately. Before a computer is left unattended, ensure that the electronic session has been terminated by logging off any electronic medical record software. Finally, a coding professional should be familiar with the HIPAA policies and procedures that govern a covered entity and participate in an annual HIPAA compliance training program.

Deliberate and Unintentional HIPAA Violations

An example of a **deliberate** violation would be failure to notify an affected individual of a breach within 60 days. A case like this involving 12 hospitals in the Virginia and North Carolina area actually occurred. After mailing 577 letters to the wrong addresses that contained PHI, Sentara Hospitals refused to notify each of the individual patients of the breach. As a result, fines totaling $2.175 million were incurred and Sentara Hospitals were subject to 2 years of monitoring. An example of an **unintentional** violation would be the theft of a laptop that contained unencrypted ePHI. In 2009, a broken laptop containing unencrypted data on 13,000 patients treated at Stanford was stolen, leading to a $20 million lawsuit against the hospital.

False Claims Act

The False Claims Act is a United States federal law that prohibits any person or entity from knowingly reporting a false or fraudulent claim to Medicare or Medicaid to obtain payment. For example, reporting and requesting reimbursement for prescription drugs or services that were not dispensed is considered a violation of the False Claims Act. The penalties include fines of up to $11,000 per claim and/or imprisonment. If an employee is aware of this type of activity taking place, they may file a whistleblower complaint at https://www.osha.gov/whistleblower/WBComplaint.html. Under the qui tam whistleblower provision, an employee is not only protected from employer reprisal, but he or she may also receive a monetary reward if the entity is found guilty.

Anti-Kickback Statute

The federal Anti-Kickback Statute prohibits physicians and entities from offering, paying, or soliciting to obtain federal healthcare business and/or patient referrals. As stated by the OIG, this includes not just monetary payments, but also "free rent, expensive hotel stays and meals, and excessive compensation for medical directorships or consultancies." Kickbacks in the healthcare field can lead to corruption; overutilization of services, durable medical equipment, or prescriptions; and unnecessary costs to the Medicare and Medicaid programs. Noncompliance to the Anti-Kickback Statute may result in exclusion from Medicare and Medicaid programs, civil penalties up to $50,000 per violation, and imprisonment.

Stark Law

Under the Stark Law, otherwise known as the Physician Self-Referral Law, physicians are prohibited from referring certain designated health services that are payable by Medicare or Medicaid, to which they, or their immediate family, have a financial relationship with. Designated health services include laboratory services, therapy services, radiology services, radiation therapy services and supplies, durable medical equipment, home health services, prescription drugs, and inpatient and outpatient hospital services. For example, a physician who has ownership of a wheelchair company and routinely refers his patients to it, would be held accountable to the Stark Law. Penalties include denial and refunding of issued payments and exclusion from Medicare and Medicaid.

AHIMA's Standards of Ethical Coding

AHIMA's Standards of Ethical Coding

AHIMA's Standards of Ethical Coding are essential guidelines based on AHIMA's code of ethics. AHIMA's Standards of Ethical Coding are put in place for coding professionals, regardless of which setting they may work in or the credentials they may hold. These guidelines offer **values** and **principles** that relate to the decision-making processes of coding and the functions of workplace activities. As of December 2016, there are 11 key ethical coding principles to which AHIMA members should aspire to and by which their work can be evaluated. Also contained in its guidelines are definitions and examples of how each principle should be interpreted and implemented.

Importance

Coding professionals commonly face **complex** regulatory requirements, **confusing** documentation, and sometimes **unclear** coding policies. Without having a clear set of essential guidelines in place that all coding professionals are expected to follow and be judged by, proper coding techniques would be completely subjective and perhaps even profit based. Therefore, knowing and understanding AHIMA's Standards of Ethical Coding are essential to help guide professionals to make decisions based on principles and to ensure their commitment to the integrity of their patients and coding activities.

Applying Accurate, Complete, and Consistent Coding Practices

In order to apply accurate, complete, and consistent coding practices that are aligned with the code of ethics set forth by AHIMA, coding professionals should not only be able to support their coding selection based on medical indicators, but they should also comply with their organization's coding policies. If an internal coding policy does not exist, one should be developed to provide a basis for the work process. For example, an internal coding policy may mandate that all coding errors that arise from the result of an audit must be corrected within 30 days. An internal coding policy may also endorse the use of a coding resource, in order to maintain consistent coding throughout the organization. An internal policy promotes honest and ethical coding practices.

Gathering and Reporting Data

In the standard related to gathering and reporting data, AHIMA advises coding professionals to follow the official coding and reporting guidelines set forth by the AMA contained in the ICD-10-CM and CPT coding manuals. These guidelines are generally located after the introductory section of each book. Body-/organ-specific coding guidelines can also be located at the start of each section/chapter. Following these guidelines ensures accuracy and proper code assignments and techniques that are in accordance with AHIMA's Standards of Ethical Coding.

Avoiding Coding-Related Activities Intended to Misrepresent Data

In an effort to avoid participation in or support of any coding-related activities that are intended to misrepresent data and their meaning, a coding professional should notify management, the compliance officer, or the organization's compliance hotline when inappropriate coding practices are identified. Inappropriate coding practices would include, but are not limited to, altering or omitting diagnosis codes to receive a higher reimbursement, misrepresenting a patient's clinical condition to qualify for insurance coverage benefits, and reporting inaccurate quality outcome codes that will improve an organization's quality profile.

Facilitating, Advocating, and Collaborating with Healthcare Professionals in Search for Accurate, Complete, and Reliable Coded Data

Facilitating, advocating, and collaborating with healthcare professionals in the search for accurate, complete, and reliable coded data are essential standards in the code of ethics because they lead to more precise and proper reporting. A coding professional can show compliance by reviewing the code of ethics with physicians and other healthcare staff members. Additionally, they can host an educational session or encourage a physician to participate in one that will explain any changes in documentation requirements. In doing so, a physician will be better equipped to correctly document diagnoses, procedures, and the severity and occurrence of events leading up to an illness or injury.

Advancement of Coding Knowledge and Practice in Accordance with Code of Ethics

In order to advance coding knowledge and practice, a coding professional should meet all continuing education requirements. This includes, but is not limited to, regular participation in educational programs; researching and reading required journals, magazines and publications, and books; and maintaining AHIMA's professional certifications. In doing so, a coding professional will stay up to date with any changes related to coding, documentation, and regulatory requirements. A list of online educational resources can be found by visiting AHIMA.org and using the search engine to locate workshops, seminars, and other publications.

Maintaining Confidentiality of PHI in Accordance with Code of Ethics

Maintaining the confidentiality of PHI involves safeguards that prevent PHI from being viewed by the public. It also means that a coding professional should only access information that is required to perform their job functions. One practical way to ensure compliance to this standard is by logging off the computer when leaving the work area. Another practical suggestion is to limit conversations involving PHI to only people who can assist in resolving a coding-related inquiry. Forwarding PHI for the purpose of entertaining or jesting is a violation of AHIMA's Standards of Ethical Coding.

Workplace Behavior That Demonstrates Integrity, Fosters Trust, and Shows Commitment to Ethical and Legal Coding Practices

One primary way for a coding professional to demonstrate integrity, foster trust, and show a commitment to ethical and legal coding practices in the workplace is to act honestly. To act honestly includes, but is not limited to, being truthful about one's credentials, professional education, and experience. Another way for a coding professional to act in accordance with this standard is to demonstrate by their **actions** that they value their patients and coworkers. For example, showing all people respect regardless of their nationality, race, or education demonstrates honor and encourages others to do the same, thus creating a work environment that encompasses these three qualities.

Unethical Coding, Data Abstraction, Query Practices, and Inappropriate Activities Related to Coding

According to AHIMA's Standards of Ethical Coding, a coding professional should not "participate in, condone, or be associated with dishonesty, fraud and abuse, or deception." For example, a coder may determine that the appropriate level of service rendered by a physician is 99212 based on documentation guidelines. However, because of decreased profit margins, that physician may pressure the coder to bill at 99213, without additional proof that such a level of service was actually performed. The physician may even offer to report the service themselves. However, either situation would violate AHIMA's Standards of Ethical Coding. The coder should be firm in their resolve not to participate in coding an inappropriate level of service and may consider reporting such an encounter with the entity's compliance officer.

Refusing to Participate in Development of Coding and Coding-Related Technology Not Designed in Accordance with Requirements

By refusing to participate in the development of coding and coding-related technology that is not designed in accordance with requirements, a coding professional will only use electronic and hard-copy resources that are currently available. Electronic resources include online coding and reference material, such as AHIMA's toolkits, journals, and EncoderPro.com. Hard-copy tools include the most current HCPCS, ICD-10-CM, and CPT manuals. Bear in mind that these electronic and hard-copy resources are just tools; they do not replace a coder's professional judgment. When doubtful of how or what to report, speak with a supervisor and always consider how to best apply the principles set forth in AHIMA's Standards of Ethical Coding.

Assigning and Reporting Codes Supported by Health Record Documentation

In order for a coding professional to assign and report only codes that are clearly and consistently supported by the health record documentation, they must make practical application of the skills and knowledge they possess of the most current coding systems and official resources. For example, when a medical condition is not indexed in the classification of the ICD-10-CM manual, a coding professional should perform the extra research needed in order to confirm the most accurate code selection. When a code is indexed in the classification, a coder should still be sure to confirm it by locating it in the tabular section, as well as reviewing the conventions, guidelines, and instructional notes that go along with it.

Uniform Hospital Discharge Data Set (UHDDS)

UHDDS

The **Uniform Hospital Discharge Data Set (UHDDS)** was first implemented by HHS in 1974 as a way to collect data surrounding the inpatient hospital discharges of Medicare and Medicaid patients. Since its implementation, several revisions have been made to the initiative. Although initially these data were only reported on patients insured by Medicare and Medicaid, all insurance carriers now collect information comparable to the data required by UHDDS. Additionally, UHDDS has expanded to include not just hospitals, but also ambulatory care and long-term-care settings, such as nursing and rehabilitation communities.

Purpose

The purpose of UHDDS is to achieve comparability and uniformity in the data collected from healthcare institutions. By having a common data set that spreads across geographic areas and systems, it allows HHS to evaluate the quality and efficiency of healthcare services being rendered and to standardize the cost for which those services should be charged and paid. For example, prior to the installment of UHDDS, racial segregation was still a popularly held practice in many areas. By creating a common data set that evaluated the quality of care separate from race, hospitals were compelled to improve the overall care of every patient that they were treating.

Required Data Elements

UHDDS requires certain data elements to be abstracted from the patient record and reported to CMS for review. These data elements include:

- Patient identification
  - Medical record number
  - Name
  - Date of birth
  - Gender
  - Location of residence
  - Race
  - Ethnicity
- Provider information
  - Provider name
  - Hospital identification number
- Clinical information surrounding the patient's admission and discharge
  - The principal diagnosis and any other diagnoses
  - Procedures
  - Where the patient was discharged to
  - Dates of service
- Financial information
  - Healthcare payer
  - Total charges for services provided.

Required Data Collection

All data required by UHDDS should be documented in an individual's medical record. Any patient identification information is usually completed by the patient and is obtained prior to treatment. Next, clinical information surrounding the patient's admission and discharge is reviewed by the coding staff and matched with the appropriate ICD-10-CM and CPT codes. Each CPT code should have a cost associated with it, thus creating a total charge for the services provided. All of this information is then entered on an insurance claims form and submitted to the healthcare payer for evaluation and review.

Role of Principal Diagnosis

Under UHDDS, a principal diagnosis is the condition or disease that, after study, is determined to be the foremost reason for which the patient was admitted into the hospital or other long-term-care facility. For example, if a patient is admitted into the hospital due to uncontrolled seizures but diagnostic images later determine that the cause is a malignant neoplasm within the brain tissue, the neoplasm would be submitted as the principal diagnosis. The principal diagnosis is a required element within the UHDDS because it has a significant contribution to quality assurance and monitoring, risk-adjusted outcome studies, and reimbursement policies.

Practice Test

Multiple Choice

1. Which of the following is NOT a covered entity under the Health Insurance Portability and Accountability Act of 1996 (HIPAA) Privacy Rule?

a. The Centers for Disease Control and Prevention
b. Employer-sponsored health plan
c. Third-party billing agency
d. Healthcare provider

2. Which of the following is a risk adjustment model used by Medicare to predict health care costs and resource consumption of specific patient populations over time?

a. Risk adjustment factor (RAF)
b. Diagnosis-related groups
c. Outcome and Assessment Information Set
d. Hierarchical condition category (HCC) coding

3. Current Procedural Terminology (CPT) code 21805 is a column 2 code that has a National Correct Coding Initiative (NCCI) edit of 1 when paired with CPT code 21813. How would this be interpreted?

a. The two codes are inclusive of each other and can never be billed together.
b. If being billed together, only report one unit of each.
c. The two codes are exclusive of each other and can never be billed together.
d. The two codes can be billed together with an appropriate modifier.

4. Based on the following documentation, what would the overall medical decision making (MDM) be?

Number of diagnosis or management options: Minimal
Amount and complexity of data: Moderate
Level of risk: Moderate

a. Straightforward
b. Low complexity
c. Moderate complexity
d. High complexity

5. A patient was seen by her gynecologist to remove her intrauterine device. The removal was attempted but terminated due to excessive bleeding. How should the gynecologist report the encounter?

a. 58301-53
b. 58301-52
c. 99212-25, 58301
d. 99212, 58301-59

6. A technician performs an ultrasound of a patient's thyroid at a privately owned family practice immediately following her annual health screening. The primary care physician determines that the images are normal and advises the patient to return in one year. How should the primary care physician report the ultrasound?

a. 76536-26
b. 76536-TC
c. 76536
d. 76536-TC, 26

7. Which type of edit identifies the maximum number of units that may be reported for a CPT/HCPCS code that relates to an individual patient?

a. Medically unlikely edits
b. Add-on-code edits
c. Correspondence edits
d. Procedure-to-procedure coding edits

8. Which statement best describes a comorbidity?

a. Two or more life-threatening illnesses occurring at the same time
b. Three or more minor injuries occurring at the same time
c. Three or more chronic illnesses occurring at the same time
d. Two or more unrelated diseases occurring at the same time

9. A healthcare employee happens to meet a well-known actor during a lunch break. The employee takes a photo and shares it with his coworkers and social media. Which AHIMA Standard(s) of Ethical Coding has been violated?

a. Protect privacy and confidentiality; protect personal health information; and use technology, data, and information resources in the way they are intended.
b. Respect the dignity of every person, put the welfare of persons before self-interest.
c. Refuse to participate in unethical practices, privacy and confidentiality, respect the dignity of every person.
d. None, the act was unintentional.

10. The smoking status of a patient should generally be found in which section of a medical record?

a. Chief complaint
b. Plan
c. Examination
d. Social history

11. Which of the following is not a data element required by the Uniform Hospital Discharge Data Set (UHDDS)?

a. Location of residence
b. Provider name
c. Family history
d. Total charges for services rendered

12. A hospital director repeatedly refuses to accept residents due to a tight budget that limits training time for students. Which AHIMA Standard(s) of Ethical Coding has been violated?

a. Put the welfare of persons before self-interest.
b. Mentor colleagues to strengthen the professional workforce.
c. Respect the worth of every person.
d. Represent the profession to the public in a positive manner.

13. A physician performs a coronary artery bypass grafting using the left internal mammary artery to the right coronary, and a saphenous vein graft to the circumflex. Which CPT code(s) would be reported?

a. 33533, 33510
b. 33534
c. 33533, 33517
d. 35600, 33517

14. A patient is seen in the emergency room with second- and third-degree burns on the right hand, and second-degree burns on the left hand after being exposed to paint thinner. After a comprehensive physical examination reveals that approximately 4% of the body is affected, the physician begins preventative treatment by debriding the nonviable tissue, cleansing the areas, and applying gauze. The patient is discharged and advised to return if experiencing symptoms that indicate an infection. What CPT and International Classification of Diseases, Tenth Revision, Clinical Modification (ICD-10-CM) codes should be reported for this encounter?

a. 99283-25, 16020, T23.701A, T23.601A, T23.602A, T65.6X4A
b. 99283-25, 16020, T23.701A, T23.602A, T65.6X1A
c. 99283, T23.701A, T23.601A, T23.602A, T65.6X4A
d. 16020, T23.701A, T23.602A, T65.6X1A

15. The UHDDS defines a principal diagnosis as ______________.

a. the condition established after study to be the foremost reason for which the patient was admitted
b. the condition, sign, and/or symptom with which the patient presented and was admitted
c. the admitting physician's initial diagnosis of the patient
d. the condition that has the highest rate of mortality for the patient upon admission

16. A 62-year-old patient is admitted into observational care after a comprehensive history and exam confirms tuberculosis. He has a medical history of being human immunodeficiency virus (HIV)-positive. How should this be reported?

a. 99236, A15.9, B20
b. 99236, B20, A15.9
c. 99235, B20, A15.9
d. 99235, A15.9, B20

17. Hospital-acquired conditions (HACs) may appear up to ___ hours after a person is discharged from an inpatient hospital or facility stay.

a. 72 hours
b. 24 hours
c. 48 hours
d. 120 hours

18. Which of the following ICD-10-CM codes are exempt from present on admission (POA) indicators?

a. I69.120
b. E05.21
c. K92.2
d. O12.03

19. A patient is admitted to the hospital due to uncontrolled seizures, but diagnostic images later determine that the cause is a malignant neoplasm within the brain tissue. How should the discharge be reported if 30 minutes were spent counseling and coordinating the care of the patient?

a. 99217, C71.9, G40.909
b. 99217, R56.9, C71.9
c. 99238, G40.909, C71.9
d. 99238, C71.9

20. Which admission indicator was created so that chronic and comorbid conditions could be differentiated from those that developed during a patient's hospital stay?

a. HCC
b. DRG
c. IPPS
d. POA

21. As of April 1, 2020, CPT code 69990 (Microsurgical techniques, requiring use of operating microscope) may be reported in conjunction with CPT code 61304 (Craniectomy or craniotomy, exploratory; supratentorial). This is an example of which type of edit?

a. Medically unlikely edits
b. Add-on code edits
c. Correspondence edits
d. Procedure-to-procedure coding edits

22. Coded clinical data are used for all of the following, EXCEPT:

a. Predict potential health diseases
b. Identify fraudulent habits
c. Track public health and risks
d. Measure the quality, safety, and efficacy of care

23. An 88-year-old male patient is seen in the emergency room with complaints of pain and bleeding on his lower back. The patient reports little to no physical activity throughout the day because he gets tired easily. A physical exam reveals a deep tissue ulcer on the coccyx. The patient is admitted and given antibiotics intravenously. Should the physician be queried?

a. No, report ICD-10-CM code L98.498.
b. No, report ICD-10-CM code K27.4.
c. Yes, the physician should be queried on whether the coccyx should be coded to the buttock.
d. Yes, the physician should be queried if the ulcer is due to constant pressure.

24. All of the following are common comorbidities to hypertension EXCEPT which of the following?

a. Cataracts
b. Congestive heart failure
c. Chronic kidney disease
d. Dyslipidemia

25. Which of the following is NOT considered a global surgical package postoperative period under the Medicare Physician Fee Schedule Look-Up Tool?

a. Zero days
b. Ten days
c. Thirty days
d. Ninety days

26. Which law prohibits physicians and entities from offering expensive hotel stays in return for patient referrals?

a. The Physician Self-Referral Law
b. The Stark Law
c. The False Claims Act
d. The Anti-Kickback Statute

27. Which one of the following forms is sent to the provider by an insurance plan to identify the allowable amount of a claim?

a. Remittance advice
b. Explanation of benefits
c. Summary of reimbursement
d. Statement of receivables

28. How often is the NCCI policy manual updated?

a. Annually
b. Biannually
c. Quarterly
d. Semiannually

29. A patient requires additional surgery within the 90-day postoperative period of a knee replacement to treat an infection that has developed at the incision site. Which modifier should be appended on the procedure?

a. 24
b. 78
c. 58
d. 52

30. A 61-year-old established patient with a history of type 2 diabetes presents to his primary care physician with complaints of changes in vision and bilateral eye pain. A comprehensive eye examination reveals that the patient has cataracts. Should the physician be queried?

a. No, report ICD-10-CM code E11.36.
b. No, report ICD-10-CM code H26.9.
c. Yes, the physician should be queried if the cataracts are due to the type 2 diabetes.
d. Yes, the physician should be queried to specify what type of cataracts the patient has.

31. A 34-year-old female patient is seen by her gynecologist for her annual checkup. During the physical examination, a small lesion is noted on the left labia, which is measured and documented in the patient's chart. The patient was counseled on birth control, safe sex practices, and self-breast checks and told to follow up again in one year. Should the physician be queried?

a. No, report ICD-10-CM code Z01.419.
b. No, report ICD-10-CM codes Z01.411 and N90.89.
c. Yes, the physician should be queried as to whether the lesion is on the vulva or vagina.
d. Yes, the physician should be queried if the annual exam resulted in an abnormal or normal finding.

32. Which of the following best describes the purpose of patient safety indicators (PSIs)?

a. To reduce monetary payments of individual physicians who frequently risk patient safety
b. To provide prevention strategies aimed at improving and enforcing patient safety within the inpatient setting
c. To make the general public aware of a hospital's safety reputation in the community
d. To identify potential safety issues and generate respective hospital rankings in terms of safety

33. Which selection most accurately describes the following query: Is the sepsis due to or the result of the recent kidney infection?

a. Compliant yes-or-no query
b. Noncompliant yes-or-no query
c. Compliant open-ended query
d. Noncompliant open-ended query

34. In general, a medical record should be signed or attested to within ________ of when the services were provided.

a. 1 week
b. 3–5 days
c. 24–72 hours
d. 8 hours

35. If a patient is receiving hospice care in a physician's office, which place-of-service (POS) code should be reported on the claim?

a. 34
b. 11
c. 71
d. 62

36. A manager of a successful healthcare facility begins to take collected copayments for questionable expenses, uses the office computer to promote her own business, and up codes certain procedures to increase reimbursement. Which AHIMA Standard(s) of Ethical Coding has been violated?

a. Facilitate interdisciplinary collaboration in situations supporting ethical health information principles.
b. Refuse to participate in unethical practices; use technology, data, and information resources in the way they are intended; and protect health information.
c. Represent the profession to the public in a positive way, honorably perform health information management responsibilities, and refuse to participate in unethical practices.
d. Put the welfare of persons before self-interest; refuse to participate in unethical practices; and use technology, data, and information resources in the way they are intended to be used.

37. A patient presents with first- and second-degree burns on his left hand and a second-degree burn on his left arm caused by excessive exposure to a paint thinner. What ICD-10-CM code(s) should the physician report?

a. T23.602A, T22.60XA, T65.6X1A
b. T23.602A, T22.60XA, T23.502A, T65.6X4A
c. T23.202A, T22.20XA, T23.102A, T65.6X1A
d. T23.602A, T22.60XA, T65.6X4A

38. Which reported service may vary depending on the state it is rendered in?

a. Evaluation and management services
b. Anesthesia services
c. Pathology and laboratory services
d. Radiology services

39. Which government-run agency is responsible for creating work plans in order to assess potential oversights and risks within the healthcare field?

a. The Centers for Medicare and Medicaid
b. The Office of Inspector General
c. The Department of Financial Services
d. The Department of Health and Human Services

40. The AHIMA Standards of Ethical Coding serve six purposes. Which of the following is NOT one of them?

a. Summarize ethical principles that reflect the job's core values.
b. Establish a framework for professional behavior when faced with ethical uncertainties.
c. Encourage refusal to participate in or conceal unethical behavior.
d. Provide ethical principles by which the public can hold health information management professionals accountable.

41. A physician must create an addendum to ePHI. Which of the following should he not do?

a. Create the addendum in the same manner as previous addendums.
b. Review policies and procedures relating to addendums.
c. Print the record with the addendum for his records.
d. Create a new signature following the addendum.

42. The multiple procedure payment reduction rule applies to which of the following CPT codes?

a. 76510
b. 99213
c. 10004
d. 44500

43. If past medical, family, and social history are not documented for the evaluation and management (E/M) of a patient who requires initial hospital care, what is the highest level of service that can be coded?

a. 99221
b. 99222
c. 99233
d. 99232

44. Which of the following forms is used to make a patient aware of the potential monetary liability that they will have if their procedure is NOT likely to be covered by Medicare?

a. Payment plan contract
b. HIPAA release
c. Advance beneficiary notice
d. National coverage determination

45. Which statement best describes the purpose of the Uniform Hospital Discharge Data Set (UHDDS)?

a. To organize the quality and cost of care of patients admitted to the hospital for longer than 10 consecutive days
b. To ensure that physicians and nonclinical hospital staff observe the regulations and laws that relate to healthcare practices
c. To facilitate, advocate, and collaborate with healthcare professionals in the search for accurate and reliable coded data
d. To achieve comparability and consistency in collected data in order to evaluate the quality and efficiency of rendered services

46. A patient with a known history of hypertension presents to her physician with increased lower extremity edema and significant anasarca. The physician determines that the patient's history of acute on chronic systolic heart failure is the cause. Creatine levels were also ordered on this encounter due to the patient's stage II chronic kidney disease. What ICD-10-CM code(s) should the physician report?

a. I10, R60.0, R60.1, I50.23, N18.2
b. I13.0, I50.23, N18.2
c. I50.23, N18.2, R60.1, Z86.79
d. R60.1, I50.23, I12.9, N18.2

47. Which of the following should be confirmed prior to assuming the correct chart or creating a new one?

a. Appointment date
b. Three unique patient identifiers
c. Date of birth of the patient
d. Treating physician

48. Which of the following best describes the role of the present-on-admission (POA) guidelines?

a. To predict health care costs and resource consumption of specific patient populations over time
b. To determine how much a hospital should be paid
c. To prevent incorrect payments due to improper coding
d. To reduce unnecessary costs incurred to the Medicare program

49. A male patient experiencing hoarseness and long-term shortness of breath is seen for a follow-up visit to discuss the results of his right lung biopsy by means of a thoracotomy that occurred 3 days ago. The results confirm small cell lung cancer. The patient is given multiple treatment options, which include their success rates, risks, and side effects. The patient opts to begin radiation treatment in 2 weeks. What CPT and ICD-10-CM codes should the provider report for this encounter?

a. 99024, C34.91
b. 99212-24,25, 99024, C34.91
c. 99213-24, C34.91
d. 99214, C34.91

50. Which of the following describes therapeutic treatment?

a. A colonoscopy is performed on a patient with a family history of colorectal cancer.
b. A hysteroscopy is performed on a patient to determine the cause of vaginal bleeding.
c. A bone marrow biopsy is collected on a patient with a high white blood cell count.
d. Radiation is administered to a patient with stage IV pancreatic cancer.

51. Which of the following patients is receiving critical care services?

a. A 95-year-old male is admitted to the intensive care unit for monitoring after a stent was placed to treat a blocked blood vessel in the heart.
b. A 79-year-old male with a history of anemia is given a blood transfusion following a severe gastrointestinal hemorrhage with an unknown cause.
c. A 47-year-old female is admitted for acute respiratory failure caused by aspiration pneumonia. She is intubated, sedated, and started on 50 mg of ertapenem.
d. A 32-year-old female with a history of severe asthma presents with an oxygen saturation level of less than 93. She is given oxygen therapy through a nasal cannula and is closely monitored for carbon dioxide poisoning.

52. Which of the following was adopted by the federal government as the standard for inpatient healthcare data?

a. POA
b. OPPS
c. UHDDS
d. RBRVS

53. How is data for the UHDDS collected?

a. By submitting statistical data through CMS.gov
b. By reviewing inpatient claim submissions
c. Through annual audits
d. By submitting statistical data to the Department of Health and Human Services

54. A patient with a history of type 1 diabetes is admitted to the hospital and later develops hyperglycemia. What ICD-10-CM code(s) should the physician report if the POA indicator is N?

a. E10.69, R73.9
b. E10.9, R73.9
c. E10.65
d. R73.9

55. Which of the following is NOT a violation of HIPAA?

a. An encrypted laptop is stolen from a physician's vehicle.
b. A hospital with a multilayered cybersecurity defense experiences a data breach by a cybercriminal.
c. An office fails to perform a risk assessment of electronic health information.
d. An employee drops off patient records on a physician's porch.

56. Which service would NOT be covered under Medicare Part A?

a. Inpatient hospital care
b. Home health service
c. Observation hospital care
d. Hospice care

57. A low-risk obstetrical patient is told to come in for weekly ultrasounds in her first trimester. This is an example of what?

a. Waste
b. Abuse
c. Fraud
d. Misuse

58. A patient is seen by her primary care physician for a severe allergic reaction to strawberries. The physician administers 0.5 mg of epinephrine subcutaneously. What code(s) should the physician report?

a. J0171 (5 units)
b. 99212-25, J0171 (5 units)
c. 99213, J0171
d. 96372, J0171 (5 units)

59. Which four organizations, known collectively as the Cooperating Parties, are responsible for the official ICD-10-CM guidelines?

a. The American Health Information Management Association (AHIMA), the American Academy of Professional Coders (AAPC), the Centers for Medicare & Medicaid Services (CMS), and the American Medical Association (AMA)
b. AHIMA, AAPC, CMS, and the Medical Library Association
c. AMA, The American Hospital Association (AHA), CMS, and the National Center for Health Statistics
d. AHA, AHIMA, CMS, and the National Center for Health Statistics

60. A 27-year-old new patient presents for an annual preventative visit. The visit is normal; however, the physician spends an additional 20 minutes counseling the patient on their type 2 diabetes controlled with diet and metformin. How should the physician report his services?

a. 99385-25, 99202
b. 99385, 99213-25
c. 99385-25, 99213
d. 99385, 99202-25

61. All of the following are repercussions of a HIPAA violation, EXCEPT:

a. Fines of up to $50,000 per violation
b. Civil penalties
c. Prison sentences up to 15 years
d. Employee dismissal

62. Which CPT and ICD-10-CM codes would be used to report the removal of the appendix through an abdominal incision due to metastatic colon malignancy?

a. 44970, C18.9, C78.5
b. 44950, C78.5, C18.9
c. 44970, C78.5
d. 44950, C78.5

63. An AHIMA member copies information found in an AHIMA journal and publishes it as his own, making only a couple of slight changes. Which AHIMA Standard(s) of Ethical Coding has been violated?

a. Use technology, data, and information resources in the way they are intended and advocate for appropriate uses of information resources across the healthcare ecosystem.
b. Represent the profession to the public in a positive manner, and respect the dignity of every person.
c. State truthfully one's credentials, and refuse to participate in unethical practices.
d. Put the welfare of persons before self-interest.

64. Which healthcare staff has the most common health record discrepancies?

a. Registration
b. Physicians
c. Nurses
d. Coders

65. A patient is admitted into the hospital due to uncontrolled seizures. Diagnostic images later determine that the cause is a malignant neoplasm within the brain tissue. Which ICD-10-CM code should be principally listed as the reason for admission?

a. C71.9
b. C71.7
c. R56.9
d. G40.909

66. Why is it so important to accurately code comorbidities?

a. To optimize patient outcomes
b. To predict risk and associated healthcare costs
c. To educate physicians
d. To rectify conflicting documentation

67. Electronic medical record features, such as copy and paste, autofill, and pulling information forward, may also be referred to as what?

a. Templates
b. Paper trails
c. Addendums
d. Cloning

68. Who is responsible for designating the severity levels of comorbidities?

a. The Department of Financial Services
b. The Office of Inspector General
c. The Centers for Medicare & Medicaid Services (CMS)
d. The Department of Health and Human Services

69. A 63-year-old male patient presents for a routine colonoscopy. During the procedure, a polyp is discovered and removed. What code(s) should the physician report?

a. 45380, Z12.11, K63.5
b. 45380, K63.5
c. 45380, D12.9
d. 45378, 45380-59, D12.9, Z12.11

70. Which payment system uses a fee schedule based on the cost of the physician's work, practice expense, professional liability insurance, and geographical location of where the services were rendered?

a. Resource-based relative value scale
b. Outpatient Prospective Payment System
c. Revenue cycle
d. Outbound provider payment mechanism

71. A physician spends approximately 20 minutes with a patient, 50% of which was spent counseling on treatment options for a keloid scar resulting from a second-degree burn to the cheek. What CPT and ICD-10-CM codes should the physician report?

a. 99213, L91.0, T20.26XS
b. 99213, L91.0, T20.26XD
c. 99214, L91.0, T20.26XD
d. 99214, L91.0, T20.26XS

72. Which of the following statements is considered an appropriate physician attestation?

a. Patient was seen and evaluated.
b. I independently evaluated the patient and agree with the resident's plan of care.
c. I discussed the case with the resident and agree with their evaluation.
d. Rounded, reviewed, and agree.

73. A patient presents to a radiology facility for an x-ray of the left shoulder after colliding with another player during a soccer game two weeks ago. The x-ray was done and is negative for any fractures or breaks. The interpreting physician refers the patient to physical therapy for pain. What diagnosis codes should the physician write on the referral?

a. M25.512, W03.XXXA, Y92.322
b. M25.512, S40.912D, W03.XXXD, Y92.322
c. S40.912A, W03.XXXA, Y92.322
d. S40.912D, W03.XXXD, Y92.322

74. Which of the following is not a designated comorbidity severity level?

a. HCC
b. MCC
c. Non-CC
d. CC

75. A 22-year-old patient is seen at an urgent care facility with complaints of difficulty breathing and body chills. A physical exam reveals that she has a fever and congestion in her chest. A sputum culture is collected and tests positive for bacteria. The patient is prescribed levofloxacin and told to follow up if the symptoms persist. Should the physician be queried?

a. No, report ICD-10-CM code B96.89.
b. No, report the patient's signs and symptoms.
c. Yes, the physician should be queried to provide a diagnosis that would encompass the patient's symptoms.
d. Yes, the physician should be queried if the patient has pneumonia.

76. Assign the appropriate CPT code(s) for the following ultrasound report:

Fetal Biometry

BPD	92.9 mm
OFD	116.5 mm
HC	331.7 mm
AC	319.5 mm
Femur	67.3 mm
EFW	2,810 g
AFI	25.2 cm

Biophysical Profile (BPP): 8/8

2	Fetal breathing movements
2	Gross body movements
2	Fetal tone
2	Amniotic fluid volume

Nonstress test (NST) 11:12 am–11:47 am

The BPP and NST are reassuring, as described above. The biometry is consistent with 33 weeks 5 days of gestation. Follow up for weekly testing and serial growth ultrasounds every 3 to 4 weeks.

a. 76815, 76816, 76819, 59025
b. 76815, 76816, 76818
c. 76816, 76819, 59025
d. 76818, 76816

77. Many payers reduce reimbursement by up to 50% for procedures with which of the following modifiers?

a. 51
b. 59
c. 53
d. 58

78. In which scenario should POA indicator W be reported?

a. A patient with a history of chronic obstructive pulmonary disease develops a flare-up after she is admitted.
b. A breast abscess is discovered when an obstetric patient attempts to breastfeed after the delivery of her child.
c. A patient is admitted with suspected autoimmune thyroiditis.
d. A laceration occurs during the delivery of a fetus.

79. Which four elements must be documented to report a consultation?

a. The reason for the consultation, the time spent discussing alternative treatment options, the name of the patient's primary care physician, and a written report of the physician's physical findings
b. Which family member requested the consultation, alternative treatment options, an MDM of moderate complexity, and a written report communicated to the patient's primary care physician
c. Documentation of assumption of care, who requested the consultation, the reason why a consultation was requested, and the physician's professional opinion
d. Who requested the consultation, the reason why a consultation was requested, the consulting physician's professional opinion, and a written report communicated back to the requesting physician

80. Which CPT and ICD-10-CM codes would be used to report a posterior fusion on the L2-L5 of the spine due to degenerative disc disease?

a. 22630, 22632, M51.35
b. 22612, 22614-51, 22614-51, 22614-51, M51.37
c. 22612, 22614x2, M51.36
d. 22630, 22632-59, 22632-59, M51.37

81. By which means are HACs reported?

a. RAF score
b. NCCI edits
c. POA indicators
d. External appeals

82. Which of the following is NOT a valid reason to query a physician?

a. To determine if a condition documented in the history is active
b. To resolve conflicting documentation
c. To rectify each discrepancy
d. To clarify a documented diagnosis

83. Which selection most accurately describes the following query: Based on your clinical judgment, please provide a diagnosis that could encompass the documented findings of shortness of breath, productive cough, and a positive culture for streptococcus.

a. Compliant yes-or-no query
b. Noncompliant multiple-choice query
c. Compliant open-ended query
d. Noncompliant open-ended query

84. A patient was admitted into the hospital with symptoms of fever and difficulty breathing. Three days later, the patient is discharged with confirmed pneumonia. Which POA indicator should be reported for this encounter?

a. Y
b. N
c. U
d. 1

85. All of the following are recommended to combat health record discrepancies EXCEPT for which?

a. Adequate training
b. Policies and procedures handbook
c. Internal reporting system
d. External audits

86. A patient presents to urgent care with a temperature of 100.2, an elevated heart rate, leukocytosis, shortness of breath, and a confirmed urinary tract infection. After the provider examines the patient, the following codes are entered on the patient's claim: R50.9, R00.0, D72.829, R06.02, A41.9, and N39.0. What code(s) should be removed?

a. R50.9
b. R50.9, R00.0, and R06.02
c. R50.9, R00.0, R06.02, and D72.829
d. A41.9

87. Which selection most accurately describes the following query: The documented history of the patient reveals that the diabetes first occurred at age 10. Can the condition be further specified as type 1 or type 2?

a. Compliant yes-or-no query
b. Noncompliant yes-or-no query
c. Compliant multiple-choice query
d. Compliant open-ended query

88. Which of the following best describes the role of the NCCI?

a. To predict health care costs and resource consumption of specific patient populations over time
b. To determine how much a hospital should be paid
c. To prevent incorrect payments due to improper coding
d. To reduce unnecessary costs incurred to the Medicare program

89. Through which incentive is a physician awarded higher reimbursement rates for enhanced quality of care and improved patient outcomes?

a. Bundled payments for care improvement initiative
b. Pay-for-performance initiative
c. Quality payment program
d. Hospital readmission reduction program

90. When a breach involves 500 or more individuals, how long does a physician or entity have to notify an affected individual from the date of its discovery?

a. 60 days
b. 30 days
c. 120 days
d. 90 days

91. Which of the following is a federal system of health insurance that is monitored and administered by each state?

a. Medicaid
b. Blue Cross and Blue Shield
c. Medicare
d. The American Association of Retired Persons

92. A physician documents an expanded problem-focused history, a comprehensive examination, and a medical decision-making encounter of moderate complexity in their admission note. Which CPT code should be reported?

a. 99221
b. 99232
c. 99222
d. 99233

93. Which selection most accurately describes the following query: Please document if you agree that the patient has polycystic ovary syndrome based on the physical findings of hirsutism and ovarian cysts.

a. Compliant yes-or-no query
b. Noncompliant yes-or-no query
c. Compliant open-ended query
d. Noncompliant open-ended query

94. A physician suspects malignancy and decides to remove two lesions from the patient's back to confirm. The size of the first lesion has a diameter of 1.0 cm, and the excised diameter is 1.9 cm. The size of the second lesion has a diameter of 3.3 cm, and the excised diameter is 4.1 cm. Which CPT codes should the physician report?

a. 11406, 11402-51
b. 11406, 11402-59
c. 11402, 11406-51
d. 11402, 11406-59

95. An established 60-year-old female patient is seen for her annual well-woman exam. The physician reports normal findings and advises the patient to report in one year. If the patient's health insurance coverage is Medicare, how should this be reported?

a. 99401, Z00.00
b. 99396, Z01.419
c. 99213, Z00.00
d. G0101, Z01.419

96. A female patient with a history of para 3, gravida 2 is seen by her obstetrician-gynecologist at 32 weeks gestation for indications that include pregestational type 2 diabetes, chronic hypertension, hyperlipidemia, and advanced maternal age. How should these diagnosis codes be sequenced?

a. O99.283, E11.9, E78.5, O09.523, O10.013, Z3A.32
b. O24.113, E11.9, O10.013, O09.523, O99.283, E78.5, Z3A.32
c. O09.523, O24.113, E11.9, O10.013, O99.283, E78.5, Z3A.32
d. O10.013, I10, O24.113, O99.283, E78.5, O09.523, Z3A.32

97. A gastroenterologist submits an out-of-network claim for a member of the following plan, in which the patient has met his deductible. The allowable amount of the claim is $170. What is the member responsible for paying?

Healthy Humans Plus Plan

Primary Care	Covered at 100%
Specialist Care	Subject to Deductible
Hospital Care	Subject to Deductible
Copay	$0
In-Network Deductible	$1,600, Covered at 75%
Out-of-Network Deductible	$2,375, Covered at 55%

a. $127.50
b. $76.50
c. $93.50
d. $42.50

98. Beginning January 1, 2021, which of the following is no longer a required component to level an E/M?

a. Examination
b. MDM
c. Face-to-face time
d. Non-face-to-face time

99. A patient is seen with complaints of tremors, which are caused by the cyclosporine that the patient takes for anemia. What ICD-10-CM code(s) should be reported for the encounter?

a. R25.1, T45.4X5A, D63.9
b. D63.9, G25.1, T45.1X5A
c. G25.1, T45.1X5A, D63.9
d. G25.1, T45.4X5A, D63.9

100. Which of the following is NOT considered an HAC?

a. Central-line-associated bloodstream infection
b. Hip fracture due to a fall
c. Postoperative fungal infection
d. Diabetic foot ulcer

Medical Scenarios

Scenario #1

Urgent Care Clinic

Date: 8/05

Progress Note: A 43-year-old male patient with a history of type II diabetes presents to an urgent care clinic with right foot pain, fatigue, muscle aches, and a fever of 101.4 °F that began 5 days ago.

Physical Exam:

- Constitutional: Oriented to person, place, and time, +fever
- Musculoskeletal: + Decreased range of motion due to generalized muscle pain, no edema, absent left big toe
- Skin: Warm and dry, no rash or ulceration noted, + cellulitis on right heel
- Pulmonary/Chest: Effort is normal and breath sounds are normal, no respiratory distress
- Abdominal: Soft, bowel sounds are normal, no masses or tenderness
- Eyes: Pupils are equal, round, and reactive to light; extraocular movement is normal

Assessment: Cellulitis of the right foot.

Plan: The patient was prescribed amoxicillin and Augmentin and instructed to take 350 mg every 12 hours and follow up in 3 days.

101. The following codes are entered on the patient's claim: E11.628, L03.115, M79.671, R53.83, M79.10, R50.81, and Z79.84. Which code(s) should be removed? Select as many as is appropriate.

a. E11.628
b. L03.115
c. M79.671
d. R53.83
e. M79.10
f. R50.81
g. Z79.84
h. None

102. If the patient has been treated at this urgent care clinic within the last three years, what CPT code should be reported for this encounter?

a. 99215
b. 99214
c. 99213
d. 99212
e. 99202
f. 99203
g. 99204
h. 99205

Scenario #2

Admission Date: 1/17

Discharge Date: N/A

Admitting Diagnosis: Altered mental status, confusion

Chief Complaint: A 68-year-old male was admitted one day ago for altered mental status and confusion that began several days ago.

Past Medical History: Hydronephrosis status post two nephrostomy tubes, hypertension, chronic kidney disease stage II, hyperlipidemia, and acute on chronic heart failure with reduced ejection fraction

Physical Exam:

- General: Not oriented to time and date, appears dehydrated
- Skin: Warm, dry, no lesions, appropriate color
- Eyes/Ears/Nose: Pupils reactive, nasal septum is midline, ear canal is clear without discharge
- Throat: Not swollen, no nodules or lesions, moist and pink
- Cardiac: BP 140/100, strong pulse
- Respiratory: 20 breaths per minute, no fluid or wheezing
- Abdomen: Soft, nontender, no bruising, masses, or splenomegaly
- Genitourinary: Nephrostomy tube in place, urine appears dark and has a strong odor, no external masses, lesions, or rash noted

Impression: Patient likely has sepsis due to pseudomonas noted in the urine culture. Urinary tract infection is in doubt due to the nephrostomy tube.

Plan: Patient will continue on intravenous fluid and be given a high dose of Bactrim. Will monitor blood pressure. Patient will continue anticoagulants and Lipitor.

103. What should the principal ICD-10-CM code be for this encounter?

a. R41.82 or R41.0 — Both are equally responsible for the admission
b. B96.5
c. N39.0
d. A41.52
e. T83.512A
f. T83.512S
g. A41.9
h. I50.23

104. Which other ICD-10-CM code(s) should be reported? Select all that apply.

a. R41.82
b. I50.9
c. N39.0
d. B96.5
e. I10
f. N18.2
g. E78.5
h. I50.23
i. I13.0

105. Which CPT code should be reported for this encounter?

a. 99233
b. 99232
c. 99231
d. 99239
e. 99220
f. 99221
g. 99222
h. 99223

SCENARIO #3

Outpatient Care: Anesthesiology

Date: 9/19

Anesthesia: General

Start Time: 7:02 am

End Time: 7:47 am

Indications: This is a 58-year-old female patient who presents with a history of multiple fractures of the right lower extremity. She is essentially wheelchair bound but can stand for short periods. She states that she was getting up and attempting to stand up when she lost her balance and twisted her right leg, resulting in severe deformity and pain at the distal femur. Emergency department radiographs identified a displaced condyle fracture of the distal femur. Based on the severity of the injury, a hinge arthroplasty was recommended, and the patient, understanding the risks and complications, consented to proceed.

Checklist: Reviewed lab results, patient summary, allergies, past medical history, electrocardiogram, nursing notes, beta blocker status, medications, consultations, nothing-by-mouth status, and problem list.

Temp	97
Pulse	100
Resp.	22
SpO_2	94%
BP	86/59

Patient Location: Operating room

Indication: Continuous blood pressure monitoring

Laterality: Right

Site: Brachial

Maximal Sterile Barrier Technique: Hand washing, cap/mask, sterile gloves and dressing, sterile gel and probe over, BioPatch

Local Anesthetic: None

Prep: Chlorhexidine gluconate

Catheter Size: 20G

Catheter Length: 1¾ inch

Ultrasound-Guided: Yes

Seldinger Technique: Yes

Line Secured: Transparent dressing and tape

Events: Patient tolerated procedure well with no complications or multiple attempts

106. Which CPT code(s) should be reported for this encounter? Select all that apply.

a. 27132
b. 01214 × 3 units
c. 27437
d. 01215 × 3 units
e. 27443
f. 27447
g. 27134
h. 01402 × 3 units

107. What ICD-10-CM code(s) should be reported for this encounter? Select all that apply.

a. Z96.651
b. X50.1XXA
c. S72.411A
d. Z87.81
e. W19.XXXA
f. Z87.311
g. Z99.3
h. Z98.890

SCENARIO #4

Emergency Department Outpatient Record

Admission Date: 3/14

Discharge Date: 3/14

Disposition: Medicine unit

Admitting Diagnosis: Acute hypoxic respiratory failure, COVID-19, pneumonia, AKI, CKI III

Chief Complaint: A 72-year-old male patient complaining of difficulty breathing, cough, and fever. Spent time with granddaughter who recently tested positive for COVID-19. Patient has not been tested.

Past Medical History: Chronic kidney disease stage III

- General: Well-nourished, chronically ill appearing, + fever 101.5 °F
- Lungs: + trace basilar crackles to auscultation bilaterally, tachypneic respirations, symmetric aeration
- Eyes/Ears/Nose: Pupils midrange bilaterally, oropharynx clear with moist mucous membranes, patent airway
- Skin: Warm, dry, normal skin turgor, no acute rashes
- Psychiatric: Cooperative, normal mood and behavior
- Cardiovascular: Heart rate and rhythm are regular; no cardiac murmurs, gallops, or rubs discerned; radial pulses present and equal bilaterally
- Neurologic: Alert and oriented ×, normal speech, + weakness
- Abdomen: Soft, nondistended, nontender to palpation, no peritoneal signs

Impression: Patient has confirmed COVID-19 pneumonia, presenting with acute hypoxic respiratory failure and acute kidney failure. Patient is suspected to have sepsis due to leukocytosis and elevated prolactin levels.

Plan: Will start patient on azithromycin, ceftriaxone, and intravenous fluid at 100 cc/hour and follow up in 3 hours. 60 minutes was spent with this patient, excluding time spent on procedures.

108. Select the most appropriate procedure code(s) to describe the above scenario.

a. 99223
b. 99281
c. 99292
d. 99285
e. 94660
f. 99291
g. 99284
h. 99222

109. Which ICD-10-CM code should be principal?

a. A41.9
b. U07.1
c. J12.89
d. J96.01
e. D72.829
f. R79.89
g. N18.30
h. N17.9

110. What other ICD-10-CM codes should be reported? Select all that apply.

a. J96.01
b. J12.89
c. D72.829
d. A41.9
e. N17.9
f. R79.89
g. N18.30
h. U07.1

SCENARIO #5

Admission Date: 12/3

Discharge Date: N/A

Admission Diagnosis: Diabetic ketoacidosis

Chief Complaint: A 64-year-old female presented to the emergency department for evaluation following an episode of syncope this morning with blood sugar measurement of 26. The patient was awoken by emergency medical services and given dextrose 10% intravenously. The blood glucose in the emergency department is 76, and the patient is drinking apple juice. The patient had limited recollection of events or symptoms; however, she currently feels asymptomatic. No fevers, cough, chills, dyspnea, fatigue, or sore throat.

Past Medical History: Type 2 diabetes mellitus on Humulin R U-500 110 units, hypertension, obesity

Physical Exam:

- SpO_2 98%
- Height 5′8″
- Weight 311 lb 8 oz using a scale in the bed
- Body mass index (BMI) 46.67
- Cognitive: Alert and oriented (AAO) × 3, appears to be in no distress
- Head: Normocephalic
- Neck: Normal range of motion, supple
- Abdominal: Soft, nontender, no quadrant pain or palpable masses
- Skin: Warm and dry, no rash, drainage, or cellulitis noted on extremities or back
- Psychiatric: Normal mood and affect, thought content is normal, no signs of depression or anxiety
- Pulmonary: Effort and breath sounds are normal, no wheezing, in no apparent distress
- Cardiovascular: Heart rate, rhythm, and sound all appear normal, strong distal pulses, equal

Impression: Diabetic ketoacidosis

Plan: Due to the patient's comorbidities, I expect that this patient requires a minimum of two overnight stays to monitor ketoacidosis. Will admit and increase insulin to 150 units until a substantial rise in blood glucose is established.

111. Which CPT code should be reported for this encounter?

a. 99221
b. 99222
c. 99223
d. 99231
e. 99232
f. 99233
g. 99218
h. 99219

112. Which ICD-10-CM code(s) should be reported? Select all that apply.

a. Z79.4
b. E16.2
c. R55
d. E66.9
e. E11.10
f. I10
g. Z68.42
h. R73.09

Scenario #6

Outpatient Care: Primary care physician

Date: 7/23

Progress Note: 56-year-old established male here for annual physical. He is overall doing well at this point, really without issues or concerns. His blood test results were reviewed with him, and his levels are stable. Overall, he has been feeling very well.

Physical Exam:

BP 128/80, pulse, 92, respirations 20, height 5′9″, weight 133.8 kg, BMI 43.56

- Constitutional: Patient is alert, pleasant, and in no acute distress. Well-developed, well-nourished, +obesity
- HEENT: Atraumatic, normocephalic, extraocular muscles intact, pupils equal and reactive to light, no signs of conjunctivitis, tympanic membranes are clear without lesions, neck without lymphadenopathy, trachea midline, no carotid bruits
- Respiratory: Clear to auscultation bilaterally without any wheezes, he is moving air very well, no accessory muscles of respiration
- Cardiovascular: Normal rate, normal rhythm, no murmurs
- Gastrointestinal: Soft, nontender, and nondistended, normal active bowel sounds, no rebound or guarding
- Musculoskeletal: Patient without edema, 5+/5+ strength bilaterally in all upper and lower extremities, patient moving all extremities equally
- Psychiatric: Speech and behavior appropriate

Assessment: Physical exam with abnormal finding of obesity.

Plan: Patient counseled for 20 minutes on exercise, nutrition, and weight loss. Advised to follow up in 3 months for a weight check. Recommended Cologuard and a CT scan of his chest for screening purposes; recommended flu, shingles, and tetanus booster. Administered 0.5 mL IIV3 P/F shot intramuscularly in the office.

113. Which ICD-10-CM code(s) should be reported? Select all that apply.

a. Z01.411
b. Z00.01
c. E66.09
d. E66.3
e. Z23
f. E66.9
g. Z68.41
h. E66.8

114. Which CPT code(s) should be reported for this encounter? Select all that apply.

a. 90471
b. G0008
c. 99213
d. 96372
e. 99396
f. 99213-25
g. 99396-25
h. 90656

SCENARIO #7

Admission Date: 5/27

Discharge Date: 6/02

Admission Diagnosis: Acute respiratory failure with hypoxia

Discharge Diagnosis: Acute respiratory failure with hypoxia secondary to acute on chronic diastolic congestive heart failure

Past Medical History: Hypertension, hyperlipidemia, coronary artery disease, cerebral vascular accident

Hospital Course: The patient was admitted with complaint of significant increased swelling in her legs despite increased diuretic at home with addition of metolazone started by her cardiologist. The patient was treated with intravenous furosemide. She had greater than 9 L of fluid out during her hospitalization with her lower extremity edema being significantly improved. The patient had shortness of breath requiring oxygen but was on room air at the time of discharge. She was able to ambulate independently with a walker. She will be discharged with home nursing for close follow-up, and she will be started in the Helping Heart program.

Discharge Exam:

Blood pressure 136/69, pulse 80, temperature 99 °F, respiration rate 16, height 5′, weight 104 kg, SpO_2 95%

- General: Patient is alert, oriented, and in no acute distress
- Neck: Soft and supple, no carotid bruits, no thyromegaly
- Head, eyes, ears, nose, and throat (HEENT) exam: Normocephalic and atraumatic, pupils equally round and reactive to light, sclerae are anicteric, no conjunctivitis or subconjunctival lesions
- Abdomen: Soft, nontender and nondistended, bowel sounds are normoactive, no guarding or rebound tenderness, no palpable masses or hernias, no suprapubic tenderness
- Coronary: Regular rate and rhythm without murmurs, rubs, or gallops
- Pulmonary: Normal respiratory effort, lungs are clear to auscultation bilaterally without wheezing
- Extremities: Warm without clubbing, edema in lower extremities greatly improved
- Neurologic: Alert and oriented to person, place, and time; cranial nerves II–XII are intact; strength and sensation are grossly intact; no focal deficits

More than 30 minutes was spent counseling and coordinating the care of this patient.

115. What should the principal ICD-10-CM code be for this encounter?

a. I11.0
b. J96.01
c. E78.5
d. I50.31
e. I11.1
f. I50.33
g. I10
h. I25.10

116. Which other ICD-10-CM code(s) should be reported? Select all that apply.

a. I25.10
b. Z86.73
c. I11.0
d. I50.33
f. I10
g. E78.5
h. J96.01

117. Which CPT code should be reported for this encounter?

a. 99231
b. 99238
c. 99315
d. 99232
e. 99316
f. 99239
g. 99233
h. 99217

Scenario #8

Emergency Department Outpatient Record

Admission Date: 2/23

Discharge Date: 2/23

Disposition: Medicine unit

Admitting Diagnosis: Burns

Chief Complaint: A 35-year-old male patient complains of a burn to the left thigh caused by a fire.

Past Medical History: Diabetes

- General: AAO×3
- Skin: Significant burns measuring approximately 5 inches on the lateral portion of the left thigh; no other burns are observed
- Eyes/Ears/Nose: Pupils reactive, nasal septum is midline, canal is clear without discharge
- Throat: Not swollen, no nodules, lesions, moist and pink
- Cardiac: BP 120/99, strong pulse
- Respiratory: 30 breaths/minute, no evidence of smoke inhalation
- Abdomen: Soft, nontender, no reported quadrant pain

Impression: Approximately 4% of the body is affected by burns reaching the dermis layer of the skin; nonviable tissue needs to be removed to avoid infection.

Plan: After consent was obtained, I debrided the wound, cleansed the area, and applied a gauze on the left thigh. Patient should continue 500 mg of metformin and be monitored for hyperthermia and shock.

118. Which CPT code(s) should be reported for this encounter? Select all that apply.

a. 99283-25
b. 97602
c. 99282
d. 99282-25
e. 99284
f. 99284-25
g. 99283
h. 16020

119. Select the primary ICD-10-CM code.

a. T24.011A
b. T24.111A
c. T24.212D
d. T24.011D
e. T24.311A
f. T24.311D
g. T24.111D
h. T24.212A

120. Which additional ICD-10-CM code(s) should be reported for this encounter? Select all that apply.

a. E10.628
b. Z79.84
c. T31.10
d. Z79.4
e. E11.628
f. E11.9
g. X08.8
h. T31.0

Answer Key and Explanations

Multiple Choice

1. A: A covered entity is any person or organization that provides treatment or payment in the healthcare field. These include healthcare providers, healthcare clearinghouses, business associates such as third-party billing companies or consulting agencies, and any individual or group health plan. Public health authorities, which include state and local health departments and the Centers for Disease Control and Prevention, are not considered covered entities.

2. D: Hierarchical condition category (HCC) coding is a risk adjustment model established in 2004 to predict health care costs and resource consumption of a specific patient population over time. Costs and consumption are calculated using a risk adjustment factor (RAF) score assigned to more than 9,500 ICD-10-CM codes associated to one of the 79 HCCs. The Outcome and Assessment Information Set is a quality measurement tool used to report and improve the quality of care delivered to Medicare and Medicaid patients in the home health setting. Diagnosis-related groups (DRGs) refer to a classification system that factors in the age, gender, diagnosis, and procedures performed during a patient's inpatient hospital stay to determine how much the hospital should be paid.

3. D: Column one represents a correct code when listed next to column two. There are three edits listed with the combination of the two columns: 0, 1, and 9. Edit 0 means that the two codes should never, under any circumstance, be reported together. Edit 1 means that the procedures may be coded together with the use of a modifier. Edit 9 means that the edit does not apply.

4. C: Two of the highest three components should be used to determine the level of complexity. In this case, because the complexity of data and level of risk are moderate, the MDM is considered moderate. If the highest two components fall into different categories, the lower of the two would determine the score. This scoring method is the same for the 1995 and 1997 documentation guidelines.

5. A: Modifier 53 is used when a procedure has been discontinued, perhaps for the patient's own health. Keywords such as "terminated" and "aborted" are clear indicators of a discontinued procedure. Modifier 52 describes services that are rendered but reduced. Key phrases such as "part of procedure eliminated" are clear indicators of a reduced service. Additionally, there is not enough medical evidence to support a separately billed evaluation and management (E/M) code because the patient was only seen for the removal of an intrauterine device.

6. C: Modifier 26 is used to indicate that only the professional component of a service was rendered. In this scenario, modifier 26 would be appended if the primary care physician only interpreted the images of the ultrasound that was done off site. Modifier TC is used to indicate that only the technical component of a service was rendered. In this scenario, modifier TC would be appended if the family practice performed the ultrasound but then forwarded the images to another practice for interpretation. On the other hand, when a physician either owns or is employed by an entity that owns the equipment and interprets the results, only the procedure should be billed without any modifier.

7. A: Add-on code edits are used when a service or procedure follows another primary CPT/HCPCS code. Procedure-to-procedure coding edits alert the provider of two procedures that are mutually exclusive to each other, meaning it would be unreasonable to have performed these two procedures or services during the same session.

8. D: A comorbidity occurs when a patient has two or more unrelated diseases or disorders occurring at the same time.

9. A: Even though the act may have been unintentional, the following principles were violated:

- AHIMA principle 1: *Advocate, uphold, and defend the consumer's right to privacy and the doctrine of confidentiality in the use and disclosure of information.* The employee did not respect the patient's right to privacy by sharing the photo to social media and with other coworkers.
- AHIMA principle 3: *Preserve, protect, and secure personal health information in any form or medium and hold in the highest regard health information and other information of a confidential nature obtained in an official capacity, taking into account the applicable statutes and regulations.* The employee did not protect the patient's health information (e.g., where they are receiving treatment) by sharing the photo to social media.
- AHIMA principle 5: *Use technology, data, and information resources in the way they are intended to be used.* By sharing a picture to social media, the employee is using secure data outside the scope of their job.

10. D: Although documentation methods vary for each physician, the medical record will generally begin with the patient's chief complaint, which is the reason for the visit. Following that would be a patient's past, social, and family history, including whether or not the patient smokes or drinks, and other risk factors that he or she may be susceptible to. Next is a physical exam, usually focused on the patient's chief complaint. Once the physician has collected an intake and has examined the patient, a diagnosis and plan can be made as to how to address the patient's concerns, illness, and/or injury.

11. C: The UHDDS requires certain data elements to be abstracted from the patient record and reported for review. These include:

- Patient identification
  - Medical record number
  - Name
  - Date of birth
  - Gender
  - Location of residence
  - Race
  - Ethnicity
- Provider information
  - Provider name
  - Hospital identification number
- Clinical information surrounding the patient's admission and discharge
  - Principal and other diagnoses
  - Procedures
  - Where the patient was discharged to
  - Dates of service

- Financial information
    - Healthcare payer
- Total charges for services provided

12. B: The seventh principle includes providing "directed practice opportunities for students" (AHIMA Standard of Ethical Coding 7.1), which the hospital director is refusing to be a part of.

13. C: Arterial grafts are reported with CPT codes 33533–33536. Because only the internal mammary artery was used, the appropriate option would be the single arterial graft (CPT code 33533). Additionally, CPT code 33517 should be reported as an add-on code to report the obtaining and grafting of the saphenous vein graft.

14. B: When billing for physician services in the emergency room, it is appropriate to also report a stand-alone E/M when the documentation supports its necessity in determining the need for appropriate treatment. Additionally, when multiple burns on the same anatomic location and laterality are being treated, identify and code only the highest degree of burn recorded in the assessment. In this scenario, only the third-degree burns on the right hand and second-degree burns on the left hand would be reported. Finally, like poisoning codes, toxic effect codes specify the intent (accidental, self-harm, assault, or undetermined). When the intent is not documented, ICD-10-CM guidelines stipulate that "accidental" should be used as the default, which in this scenario would be T65.6X1A (Toxic effect of paints and dyes, not elsewhere classified, accidental, initial encounter).

15. A: A principal diagnosis is the condition or disease that, after study, is determined to be the foremost reason for which the patient was admitted into the hospital or other long-term-care facility. A principal diagnosis is a required element within the UHDDS because it has a significant contribution to quality assurance and monitoring, risk-adjusted outcome studies, and reimbursement policies.

16. B: All observation codes (99234–99236) include a comprehensive history and exam. The MDM of this condition is considered high (the number of diagnoses and risk of complication), making the CPT code 99236, as opposed to CPT code 99235. Even though tuberculosis is the reason for the admission, ICD-10-CM guidelines stipulate that a confirmed HIV diagnosis takes precedence in sequencing when the reason for admission is HIV-related. HIV-related conditions are identified in the ICD-10-CM manual with a black "HIV" symbol.

17. A: Hospital-acquired conditions (HACs) may appear up to 72 hours after a patient has been discharged or within 30 days of an operation. Patients cannot be billed for care related to an HAC, and most health insurance plans will not pay for their treatment.

18. A: Conditions arising as a sequela of another disease, newborns affected by maternal illnesses and/or injuries, and congenital malformations are all exempt from POA indicators because they may occur some time after a patient's admission but are usually not preventable by hospital staff and physicians.

19. D: The appropriate CPT codes for a hospital discharge following an inpatient admission are 99238–99239. CPT code 99217 describes discharge services from outpatient hospital observation status. The principal diagnosis code should always be the underlying illness and/or disease that necessitated the treatment. In this scenario, the brain malignancy is the underlying reason for the seizures and should therefore be reported as the primary code. Because seizures are a common symptom of a brain malignancy, R56.9 (Unspecified convulsions) should not be reported.

20. D: Present-on-admission (POA) indicators were created so that hospitals could differentiate chronic and comorbid conditions from those that developed during an inpatient admission. These indicators were created in lieu of the implementation of HACs, which affected payment and quality ratings.

21. B: The first step is to locate CPT code 69990 in the CPT manual. The description of the code indicates that the procedure is an add-on code; therefore, the type of edit that would encompass it is an add-on code edit. Medically unlikely edits are used to identify the maximum number of units that may be reported for a CPT/HCPCS code, whereas procedure-to-procedure coding edits are applied when two procedures are mutually exclusive to each other.

22. A: Coded clinical data are used to

- Set health policy
- Identify fraudulent habits within the healthcare system
- Monitor utilization of resources and design the way it is distributed
- Perform research, studies, and trials
- Design payment systems
- Provide data regarding the costs and quality of treatment options to the public
- Follow public health
- Measure the quality, safety, and efficacy of the care being given
- Assist in improving clinical performance

23. D: In order to select the most specific and accurate diagnosis, further specification is needed to determine the type of ulcer that the patient has. Because the physician documented "little to no physical activity" and bedsores are the leading cause of ulcers in elderly people, a query asking the physician if the ulcer is due to constant pressure is nonleading and clinically relevant.

24. A: Hypertension in a condition in which the body cannot control its high blood pressure. This damages the artery walls, leading to conditions such as heart disease, heart failure, kidney disease, and dyslipidemia, all of which rely on consistent blood flow.

25. C: CMS has created three types of global surgical packages built on the duration of the postoperative period. These are a zero-day post-operative period for endoscopies and some minor procedures, a 10-day postoperative period for other minor procedures, and a 90-day postoperative period for major procedures.

26. D: Because the Anti-Kickback Statute prohibits physicians and entities from obtaining healthcare business by means of incentives or money, it reduces corruption; overutilization of services, durable medical equipment, or prescriptions; and unnecessary costs to CMS. The Stark Law, otherwise known as the Physician Self-Referral Law, prohibits physicians from referring certain designated health services that are payable by Medicare or Medicaid to which they, or their immediate family, have a financial relationship with. The False Claims Act prohibits any person(s) or entity from knowingly reporting a false or fraudulent claim to CMS to obtain payment.

27. A: The remittance advice and explanation of benefits forms identify the allowable amount of a claim, the beneficiary responsibility, and the reasons for any charges that were denied or not paid. The difference between the two forms is that a remittance advice form is sent to the medical entity where the services were rendered, whereas an explanation of benefits form is sent directly to the beneficiary.

28. C: The Centers for Medicare & Medicaid Services (CMS) update the NCCI policy manual every quarter; it can be found by visiting the following website:

https://www.cms.gov/Medicare/Coding/NationalCorrectCodInitEd

29. B: Modifier 78 is for an unexpected return to the operating room by the same physician during the postoperative period to address a complication that has developed as a result from the initial procedure. It should be noted that the billing of a new procedure with the use of modifier 78 does not extend the original postoperative period. Modifier 24 is for use on unrelated E/M services rendered by the same physician during the postoperative period. Modifier 58 is used for a procedure that is planned to take place during the 0-, 10-, or 90-day postoperative period of the first procedure.

30. A: As a result of a chemical imbalance and accumulation of excess sorbitol in the lens, patients who have diabetes are at a higher risk of developing eye complications, such as cataracts. Because of this, a causal relationship is presumed between the two conditions, as seen in the verbiage of E11.36 (Type 2 diabetes mellitus with diabetic cataract), and the physician does not need to be queried.

31. D: Knowing whether or not the gynecological exam that was performed resulted in normal or abnormal findings is essential to choosing a correct diagnosis code. By presenting the query in a multiple-choice fashion, the physician does not feel pressured to choose one option over the other.

32. D: Patient safety indicators (PSIs) are a group of 27 quality measures that were developed by the Agency for Healthcare Research and Quality as a way to identify potential safety issues within an inpatient hospital setting, including complications and adverse events following a surgical procedure and/or childbirth. PSIs are also used to generate respective hospital rankings in terms of safety. The hospital that shows the lowest percentage improvement in terms of safety within a fiscal year faces monetary penalties and reduced reimbursement rates.

33. A: Because untreated infections, especially those originating in the urinary tract, are known to cause sepsis, this query is considered compliant. Additionally, the query is asked in a manner that allows the physician to respond with a "yes" or "no" answer. These types of queries can be used to substantiate a diagnosis found in imaging or pathology, clarify conflicts in documentation, and confirm causal relationships when the documentation lends itself to it.

34. C: In general, a medical entry should be signed or attested to within 24 to 72 hours of when the services were rendered, with some exceptions that are dependent on pathology results, transcription delays, etc. An authenticated medical record ensures the protecting and archiving of health information prior to the request for payment.

35. B: Place-of-service (POS) codes "specify the entity where service(s) were rendered." In this case, hospice care was provided in an office, which would correspond to POS 11. POS 34 refers to hospice care provided in a facility, POS 71 refers to a public health clinic that provides ambulatory medical care, and POS 62 refers to an outpatient rehabilitation facility providing services that would include physical and occupational therapy. For a list of each POS and its description, see Appendix K in the CPT manual.

36. D: The following principles were violated:

- AHIMA principle 2: *Put service and the health and welfare of persons before self-interest and conduct oneself in the practice of the profession so as to bring honor to oneself, one's peers, and to the health information management profession.*
- AHIMA principle 4: *Refuse to participate in or conceal unethical practices or procedures and report such practices.* Upcoding and stealing money that belongs to the healthcare facility is fraudulent behavior and is unethical.
- AHIMA principle 5: *Use technology, data, and information resources in the way they are intended to be used.* The manager violated this principle by using the office computer to promote her personal business.

37. A: Although an injury caused by a chemical agent is classified as a corrosion and not a burn, the coding guidelines remain the same. When multiple injuries occur at the same anatomical site, only code the injury with the highest severity. In this scenario, only the second-degree burn on the left hand and the second-degree burn on the left arm would be coded because a first-degree burn only affects the outer layer of the skin, whereas a second-degree burn involves the second layer of skin. Additionally, when determining whether the intent of the corrosion was accidental or undetermined, bear in mind that unless the physician states otherwise, the default code should always be accidental.

38. B: When it comes to reporting the time for anesthesia services, the CPT manual advises that the start time begins when the anesthesiologist begins preparing the patient for induction and ends when the patient is safely placed under postoperative supervision. However, it also adds that time "may be reported as is customary in the local area." Other variations may occur with some states that recognize anesthesia assistants and others that do not.

39. B: Each year, the Office of Inspector General creates various projects, known as work plans, which help detect and combat waste, fraud, and abuse in the medical system. The Office of Inspector General's workplans can be reviewed on their website and allow coding professionals and physicians to fix their own unintended errors before becoming the target of an audit.

40. C: The six purposes of the AHIMA Code of Ethics are

- Promote high standards of the health information management practice.
- Summarize ethical principles that reflect the job's core values.
- Establish a set of ethical principles to be used to help guide decision making and the actions that follow.
- Establish a framework for professional behavior when faced with ethical uncertainties.
- Provide ethical principles by which the public can hold health information management professionals accountable.
- Mentor those who may be new to the ethical principles and values involved in the health information management field.

41. C: If a physician is transcribing reports within the electronic health record system, he/she should not print the record. Doing so risks exposing ePHI and violating HIPAA if the document is not dealt with carefully. When creating an addendum, a physician should review the company's policies and procedures handbook as it relates to addendums, create the addendums consistently (e.g., always creating them at the bottom of the note), and always re-sign the note when the addendum is completed.

42. A: Typically, under the multiple procedure payment reduction rule, the primary procedure will be reimbursed at 100% of the allowable amount and all secondary procedures will be paid at a lesser amount, usually 25% or 50% of the allowable amount. However, the multiple procedure payment reduction rule does have exceptions in which no reduction is taken, including significant and separately identifiable E/M services (e.g., CPT code 99213), add-on codes (e.g., CPT code 10004), and modifier 51 exempt codes (e.g., 44500).

43. C: In order to report CPT codes 99221–99223, the physician must document a detailed or comprehensive history intake, which must include the patient's past medical, family, and social history. If these documentation requirements cannot be met, CPT guidelines advise deferring to subsequent hospital care codes, which do not require a history intake if the documentation requirements are met for the examination and medical decision-making portions of the note.

44. C: An advance beneficiary notice can be given to a beneficiary when a service is expected to be denied by Medicare Part A or Part B; however, Medicare requires the advance beneficiary notice to be given to the beneficiary far enough in advance for them to review their medical options and make an informed decision. The National Coverage Determination is a reference guide for physicians to determine which services are covered by Medicare. A HIPAA release is a form that must be signed by the patient prior to the release of medical records, and it can be revoked at any time.

45. D: The UHDDS was implemented in 1974 by the Department of Health and Human Services as a way to collect data surrounding the inpatient hospital discharges of patients. The purpose of UHDDS is to achieve comparability and uniformity of the data collected in order to evaluate the quality and efficiency of healthcare services being rendered and standardize the cost for which those services should be charged and paid.

46. B: The primary diagnosis is the underlying condition for which treatment is being given. In this scenario, the physician has documented that heart failure is the root illness for which the patient is exhibiting symptoms. However, when coding heart failure, the ICD-10-CM manual advises to report ICD-10-CM code I11.0 (Heart failure due to hypertension) or I13.0 (Heart failure due to hypertension with chronic kidney disease) as primary. Although the physician does not explicitly state that the heart failure is "due to" hypertension or that the patient has hypertension "with" chronic kidney disease, chapter-specific guidelines instruct coders to assume that a causal relationship exists between these conditions, unless the physician documents that they are unrelated. The codes R60.0 (Localized edema) and R60.1 (Generalized edema) represent symptoms and would not be reported in lieu of a confirmed diagnosis.

47. B: Patient identifiers are required by HIPAA in order to maintain and protect a person's private health information. A patient identifier may include, but is not limited to, special alerts when accessing an electronic health record (EHR), a medical identification number, and/or confirming the patient's date of birth and full name with the patient. Confirming at least three unique identifiers prevents duplicate charts and helps deter the creation of multiple records.

48. D: In 2007, the United States government implemented present-on-admission (POA) guidelines as a way to reduce unnecessary costs incurred to the Medicare program. Under these guidelines, general acute care hospitals and facilities became responsible for differentiating illnesses and/or injuries that an individual presented with upon their admission, from those that developed later during his or her inpatient stay. POA guidelines are reported by means of one of five indicators attached to the principal and secondary diagnoses of a claim.

49. B: The postoperative period for the patient's thoracotomy procedure with a biopsy (CPT codes 32096–32098) is 90 days. A postoperative period is the time frame given from the day a procedure occurred, for the provider to address biopsy results, follow-up incisional care, and any postoperative-related complications without incurring additional charges to the patient. Because the patient was provided with his biopsy results within the 90-day postoperative period, CPT code 99024 (postoperative follow-up visit) should be reported. However, because the provider also discussed treatment options for the condition for which the procedure was performed, an E/M should also be reported. Modifiers 24 and 25 are both appended to indicate that a separately identifiable service was given during the postoperative time period of a procedure. The ICD-10-CM crosswalk for a malignant neoplasm of the right lung is C34.91.

50. D: A therapeutic procedure is one that is aimed at treating an already established disease or condition, which in this scenario would be stage IV pancreatic cancer. A colonoscopy describes a screening procedure, which is considered routine based on a patient's age and/or family history. A hysteroscopy and bone marrow biopsy are diagnostic procedures that are done with the intention of ruling out or determining a diagnosis based on the images or findings obtained from the procedure. Usually, the patient will exhibit signs or symptoms that deem the procedure to be medically necessary.

51. C: Critical care describes high-complexity MDM in the care of a patient who has a life-threatening condition. This would include endotracheal tube insertion, cardiac defibrillation, fluid administration for shock, and administration of the drug Narcan. Administering oxygen via a nasal cannula, transfusing blood, and routine and postoperative care are not considered critical care.

52. C: The Uniform Hospital Discharge Data Set (UHDDS) was adopted by the federal government as the standard for collecting healthcare data. By providing a list of data elements that are required when submitting a claim, the quality and efficiency of healthcare services being rendered can more easily be evaluated and the costs for which those services should be paid can be standardized. Present on admission (POA) is a type of guideline used to differentiate illnesses and/or injuries that a patient presented with upon their admission from those that developed later during their inpatient stay. The resource-based relative value scale (RBRVS) is a payment system calculated by factoring the cost of the physician's work, practice expense, professional liability insurance, and geographical location. The outpatient prospective payment system (OPPS) is a payment system designed to promote the predictability of payment, promote consistency, and encourage the quality of care given to Medicare patients receiving outpatient services in a hospital setting.

53. B: All of the data required by UHDDS that should be documented in an individual's medical record is reviewed and reported by the coding staff and matched with the appropriate ICD-10-CM and CPT codes. Each CPT code should have a cost associated with it, thus creating a total charge for the services provided. All of this information is then entered on an insurance claim form and is submitted to the healthcare payer for evaluation and review. This information is next collected by UHDDS to evaluate the quality and efficiency of healthcare services being rendered and to standardize the cost for which those services should be charged and paid.

54. C: When an illness or disease is POA, but a manifestation or complication of the disease presents itself during an inpatient stay, the combination ICD-10-CM code should always be reported. POA guidelines stipulate that if both conditions in the combination code are POA, the POA indicator should be Y. On the other hand, if the patient only presents with the one disease, in this case the type 1 diabetes mellitus, and later develops an associated complication, the POA indicator should be N.

55. B: HIPAA is in place to reduce the associated risk of a potential violation or breach. Although a breach has occurred in this scenario, HIPAA was not violated because the hospital took appropriate preventative measures. High-risk behaviors, such as leaving a laptop in an unattended vehicle or leaving medical records outside, allow opportunities for an unauthorized individual to access protected health information. Finally, a medical practice is required by HIPAA to perform a risk analysis of electronic health information and rectify any issues immediately.

56. C: Observation hospital care is provided to patients who are not sick enough to be admitted. Therefore, this type of care is considered outpatient and is covered under Medicare Part B.

57. A: Because the patient is not at risk and most fetal organs are not developed and/or cannot be visualized in the first trimester, weekly ultrasounds are considered wasteful and an unnecessary cost to health insurance plans. Fraud is knowingly and willfully obtaining, or attempting to obtain, money by means of false pretenses from any healthcare benefit program. Abuse is similar to fraud, with the exception that the intent is not, or cannot, be proved to be willful or knowing.

58. D: HCPCS Level II code J0171 can be found by either reviewing section J in the manual, "Drugs administered other than oral method" or by locating epinephrine in Appendix 1 in the manual, "Table of Drugs." Because 0.5 mg of epinephrine was administered, and each unit of code J0171 represents only 0.1 mg of the drug, five units should be reported. The subcutaneous injection is reported with CPT code 96372, which includes an inherent E/M component unless the physician goes beyond such services.

59. D: The four organizations responsible for the official sources of coding guidelines and conventions found in the ICD-10-CM manual are AHA, AHIMA, CMS, and the National Center for Health Statistics.

Although the official guidelines can be located in the introduction of the manual, each organization publishes its own individual resources to help its members understand relevant coding advice.

60. D: Modifier 25 is a CPT modifier that is appended on a "significant, separately identifiable evaluation and management service by the same physician" on the same day of another procedure or service. In this scenario, because the patient presented for an annual, the significant and separately identifiable service is the evaluation and management of the type 2 diabetes. When selecting the CPT codes, keep in mind that they should each reflect that the patient is new to the practice.

61. C: A covered entity who violates HIPAA may be subject to employee dismissal, fines ranging from $100 to $50,000 per violation, civil penalties, prison sentences of up to 10 years, or a combination of these.

62. B: An appendectomy for an appendix that has not ruptured is reported with CPT code 44950. CPT code 44970 is used when the documentation specifically states that the procedure was done laparoscopically versus through an abdominal incision. ICD-10-CM guidelines state that when treatment is directed only to the secondary site of malignancy, code that malignancy as principal, followed by the primary cancer.

63. D: This second principle includes taking "responsibility and credit, including authorship credit, only for work one actually performs" (AHIMA Standard of Ethical Coding 2.5). The AHIMA member dishonestly took credit for the work of someone else.

64. A: Oftentimes, registration staff are pressured to obtain a patient's information within a certain time frame, leading to the entering or obtaining of misinformation. A high turnover rate may also cause some staff to lack the knowledge needed to complete assigned tasks correctly. Oftentimes, these errors are not corrected until after the patient is discharged, resulting in health insurance plan denials and/or delayed payments.

65. A: A principal diagnosis is the condition or disease that, after study, is determined to be the foremost reason for which the patient was admitted into the hospital or other long-term-care facility. In this scenario, although the patient was admitted for seizures, studies showed that the malignancy was the underlying cause for admission. Because the location within the brain is not specified, the ICD-10-CM code should be "unspecified."

66. B: Researchers and health insurance plans rely heavily on the reported comorbidity data to predict risk and the associated healthcare costs. Medicare, for example, has been able to estimate the cost that a beneficiary will incur to the government based on their medical history. However, in order for their predictions to be accurate, the coded data must be reliable. On the other hand, coded data do not optimize patient outcomes, educate physicians, or rectify conflicting documentation.

67. D: Cloning is when the documentation for one encounter appears identical or similar to the documentation from another encounter. This can happen when a physician copies and pastes documentation, sets their templates to auto fill certain data elements, and/or pulls information forward from a previous encounter. The use of templates in and of itself does not mean that the physician is cloning documentation. Rather, the inappropriate use of this tool can lead to it.

68. C: CMS is responsible for designating and publishing the severity of ICD-10-CM codes. In doing so, it determines compensation based on associated conditions and statistical models that predict the use of resources.

69. A: A diagnostic colonoscopy without biopsies is reported with CPT code 45378. However, because a polyp was removed, CPT code 45380 should be billed instead, rather than in addition. Because the primary reason for the procedure was a screening, Z12.11 is considered the most appropriate principal code. ICD-10-CM guidelines advise that if there is an incidental finding, it may be used as an additional code.

70. A: The resource-based relative value scale (RBRVS) is a physician payment system adopted by CMS and other health insurance plans. Payments are calculated by combining the cost of the physician's work, practice expense, and professional liability insurance. The value is then multiplied by a conversion factor and adjusted based on the geographical location where the services were rendered, known as the geographical price cost index (GPCI). The resulting amount is known as a fee schedule payment. The Outpatient Prospective Payment System (OPPS) is a reimbursement method for Medicare patients receiving outpatient services, and the revenue cycle is a broad term to describe the "business side" of a practice.

71. A: When selecting an E/M based on time and the minutes fall in between two codes ranked in sequential order, the E/M closest to the actual time should be reported. In this scenario, because the midpoint of CPT codes 99213 and 99214 has not been passed, CPT code 99213 is the most accurate code selection. In choosing the appropriate seventh character for ICD-10-CM code T20.26X (Burn of second degree of forehead and cheek), remember that subsequent care is an indication that the condition is still healing, whereas a sequela is a complication or condition that arises from the original injury. A keloid scar is a sequela, or complication, arising from the original burn injury.

72. B: An attestation is a statement from a teaching physician that validates his/her review and participation of the care rendered to a patient by a medical student, resident, or fellow. According to Medicare, a teaching physician must perform or be present during the critical portions of the service rendered by a medical student, resident, or fellow and must participate in the management of the patient's care. Statements such as "Patient seen and evaluated" or "Rounded, reviewed, and agree" lack the specificity of who treated the patient. Additionally, a physician cannot prove their presence during the critical portions of the service with the statement, "I discussed the case with the resident and agree with his/her evaluation."

73. A: Because there is not a blanket code for pain in the injury section of the ICD-10-CM manual, a coder may be inclined to select S40.912 (Unspecified superficial injury to the left shoulder). However, ICD-10-CM codes should be selected based on the highest level of specificity documented. In this scenario, M25.512 (Pain in left shoulder) is the highest level of specificity; therefore, it should be the primary diagnosis reported. Subsequent codes describing why and/or how the patient came to have pain in the shoulder should be listed with the seventh character "A," indicating that the patient is receiving active treatment (i.e., diagnostic x-ray). The seventh character "D" is used to describe treatment during the recovery phase of an injury or condition.

74. A: The three severity classes of comorbidities are as follows:

- Non-CC (Non-complication/comorbidity) — a condition that does not impact the severity of the illness and the resources used
- CC (Complication/comorbidity) — a condition that has a moderate impact on the severity of the illness and the resources used
- MCC (Major complication/comorbidity) — a condition that has a major impact on severity of illness and the resources used

75. C: Although reporting signs and/or symptoms can be appropriate, the positive sputum culture suggests a more definitive diagnosis that is not currently present in the documentation and the physician should be queried to substantiate it.

76. D: The documentation supports CPT code 76816 (Ultrasound, pregnant uterus, real time with image documentation, follow up) and CPT code 76818 (Fetal biophysical profile; with non-stress testing). Although CPT code 76815 meets the documentation requirements (requiring only one of the following elements: fetal heartbeat, placental location, fetal position, and qualitative amniotic fluid volume), it is considered inclusive to CPT code 76816 and should not be billed as an additional procedure. Additionally, although CPT codes 59025 (Fetal nonstress test) and 76819 (Fetal biophysical profile) were performed, reporting them separately is considered unbundling. Finally, to ensure proper payment, sequence CPT codes in order of highest relative value units to lowest. In this scenario, CPT code 76818 has a higher reimbursement value than 76816 and should be listed first.

77. A: Modifier 51 is used when multiple procedures (excluding E/M and rehabilitation services) are performed during the same session by the same provider. Keywords like "a different procedure" or "separate from" are indicators of when modifier 51 should be appended to the secondary procedure code. Coders should be aware that when reporting secondary and tertiary procedures with modifier 51, a multiple procedure payment reduction may be applied. This means that the primary procedure will be reimbursed at 100% of the fee schedule, whereas all other procedures will be reimbursed at 25%–50% of the fee schedule.

78. B: POA indicator W is used to report an illness or condition that clinically cannot be determined whether it was POA. An incidental finding during an inpatient stay, such as a breast abscess, should be reported with POA indicator W because it would be difficult to determine when the condition was established. An exacerbation of a chronic condition or injury sustained during a hospital stay would be reported with POA indicator N because these were not present at the time of admission. Finally, any suspected, possible, or probable diagnoses documented on admission are considered present and are reported with POA indicator Y.

79. D: When documenting a consultation, the physician must include which physician requested the consultation (usually in the form of an electronic or paper referral), the reason why the consultation was requested, and a written report of their findings and/or professional opinion communicated back to the requesting physician. A consultation or second opinion occurring at the request of the patient or other family member would not be considered a consultative service.

80. C: The term "fusion" in the CPT manual index leads to "arthrodesis," which is reported with CPT codes 22612, 22614, and 22630–22634. In this scenario, the arthrodesis is performed on three levels of the lumbar spine: L2-L3, L3-L4, and L4-L5, which are reported with CPT codes 22612 and two units of 22614. Because CPT 22614 is an add-on code, no modifier should be appended on it. When choosing between ICD-10-CM codes M51.36 (Disc degermation, lumbar region) and M51.37 (Disc degeneration, lumbosacral region), bear in mind that the lumbosacral joint lies between L5 and S1, making the appropriate diagnosis code M51.36. The spinal anatomy can be found in the anatomy portion of the ICD-10-CM manual.

81. C: POA indicators serve as a way to report whether an illness and/or injury was POA into the hospital. When reporting an HAC, POA indicator N (a diagnosis was not present at the time of inpatient admission) or POA indicator 1 (the diagnosis is exempt from POA reporting) should be used on the claim form. RAF scores are used to predict health care costs and resource consumption to a specific population over time, NCCI edits are used to identify unbundled procedure codes, and external appeals are used to argue when a claim has been denied by a health insurance plan inappropriately.

82. C: A query can be used to clarify documentation and ensure accurate procedural and diagnosis coding. This includes resolving conflicting documentation, determining whether a condition documented in the history section of the medical record is still active, or seeking clarification if a documented diagnosis does not appear to be clinically supported. On the other hand, a query should never be used to increase reimbursement or rectify every discrepancy seen in a medical record.

83. C: This open-ended query is formulated based on clinical indicators in the medical record and allows the provider to express themselves freely. This type of query is used to clarify or substantiate a diagnosis based on documented results.

84. A: Although the diagnosis of pneumonia was not explicitly documented by the admitting physician, the individual's symptoms indicate that the illness existed and was POA, and it was not an illness that developed during the individual's inpatient stay, thus making the POA indicator Y. POA indicator N is used when an illness or injury is not present at the time of admission but develops during the inpatient stay. POA indicator U is used when the documentation is insufficient to determine when the condition began. Finally, POA indicator 1 is for illnesses or facilities that are exempt from the POA reporting system.

85. D: External audits are done to combat fraud, waste, and abuse. However, to combat health record discrepancies, healthcare organizations can create and implement their own policies and procedures handbook that relates directly to the appropriate use of an EHR system; provide staff with adequate training upon employment; and implement an internal reporting system that can identify, report, and correct EHR and/or EHR-related issues promptly.

86. C: Based on the codes entered, the provider has determined that the patient has sepsis (A41.9) due to a urinary tract infection (N39.0). Fever (R50.9), rapid heart rate (R00.0), and shortness of breath (R06.02) are all symptoms of both a urinary tract infection and sepsis. Additionally, the presence of elevated white blood cell counts, otherwise known as leukocytosis, is a physiological response to an acute infection and is therefore deemed to be a symptom when an infection has been confirmed. None of these four codes should be reported because ICD-10-CM guidelines stipulate that when a definitive diagnosis is present, signs and/or symptoms should not be additionally listed on the claim.

87. C: This multiple-choice query is formulated based on clinical indicators in the medical record and allows the physician to choose one or more listed diagnoses. Additionally, the query is written in a nonleading format, meaning that the physician should not feel pressured or encouraged to choose one or more choices over another.

88. C: The NCCI was created in 1994 by CMS in order to prevent incorrect payments due to improper coding. The NCCI policy manual helps providers, suppliers, and hospitals identify errors in their billing practices that help prevent payment denials and carrier-specific audits.

89. B: The pay-for-performance initiative was designed to provide an incentive to hospitals to hold physicians accountable for their actions, enhance quality of care, and improve patient outcomes. If a physician can provide evidence of compliance and improvement through reported PSIs, they are awarded with higher reimbursement rates for the services that they render. On the other hand, if little to no improvement is shown, they face monetary penalties.

90. A: When a breach involves 500 or more individuals, each affected person must be notified of the breach within 60 days of its discovery. For breaches that involve fewer than 500 individuals, an entity or physician must notify the Secretary of Health and Human Services within 60 days of the end of that calendar year. Failure to do so in both scenarios is a violation of HIPAA.

91. A: Medicare and Medicaid are public federal systems of healthcare; however, Medicaid is monitored and administered by each state and serves as a free or low-cost source of health coverage. Individuals who qualify include the following:

- Persons with low income
- Children
- Pregnant women
- Elderly adults
- Persons with disabilities

92. B: CPT codes 99221–99223 are normally used to report the initial encounter with a patient by the admitting hospital physician. However, in order to report one of these three codes, either the documentation must meet a minimum requirement of having a detailed history, detailed examination, and straightforward medical decision making, or it must meet a minimum requirement of 30 minutes spent with the patient because the expanded problem-focused history does not meet these documentation requirements. When the documentation does not meet the requirements for initial hospital care, CPT codes 99231–99233 can be reported instead because these subsequent hospital care codes only require two of the three components. In this scenario, the examination and medical decision-making support the reporting of CPT code 99232.

93. B: The query is written in a manner that allows the physician to respond with a "yes" or "no" answer. However, this query is noncompliant because polycystic ovarian syndrome is not a documented condition and is therefore leading the physician to a diagnosis.

94. B: Without a pathology report to confirm malignancy, CPT guidelines state that the excision code assumes that the lesion is benign, leading a coder to CPT codes 11400–11471. CPT code 11406 would be listed first because it is the more complex procedure, followed by CPT code 11402. Additionally, CPT guidelines stipulate that when coding more than one excision, it is appropriate to append modifier 59 to the additional, separate procedure.

95. D: Although CPT code 99396 is used to report preventative services for an established patient, Medicare requires that certain preventative visits and other services be reported with the comparable HCPCS Level II code. In this scenario, a gynecological exam (otherwise known as a well-woman exam) should be reported with HCPCS Level II code G0101 (Cervical or vaginal cancer screening; pelvic and clinical breast examination). CPT code 99401 is used to report counseling services outside of what is considered preventative, and CPT code 99213 is used to report the E/M of other illnesses. Additionally, ICD-10-CM Z01.41 (Encounter for routine gynecological exam) should be reported as the primary diagnosis on all well-woman exams.

96. C: For routine outpatient prenatal care for patients who are considered higher risk, codes from O09 should be sequenced first, followed by all of the other secondary and coexisting conditions and should be completed with the gestational age (Z3A.32). Furthermore, coders should be aware of when to use additional codes to identify specific conditions. For example, when coding ICD-10-CM code O24.113 (Preexisting type 2 diabetes mellitus), the guidelines prompt the coder to use an additional code from category E11. However, when coding ICD-10-CM code O10.013 (Preexisting essential hypertension), I10 should not be added.

97. B: The out-of-network deductible for the member is $2,375. Because this amount has been met, the insurance plan will pay 55% of the allowable amount and places the remaining 45% on the member as their responsibility. Therefore, the member is responsible for 45% of $170, or $76.50.

98. A: The American Medical Association (AMA) has outlined new office and other outpatient E/M coding guidelines that are effective January 1, 2021. Up to this point, the three components required to level a new and established office and other outpatient E/M code were history, examination, and MDM. However, these new guidelines stipulate that although a medically appropriate history and examination should be obtained, these are no longer the driving force to level an E/M. On the other hand, code selection will now be based on the total time spent by the provider, including face-to-face and non-face-to-face time, as well as the severity of the MDM.

99. C: When multiple conditions exist, the primary diagnosis code will be the foremost reason that the patient is receiving treatment. Because the patient's chief complaint is tremors caused by a medication, the primary diagnosis should be G25.1 (Drug-induced tremor). In choosing this code, the ICD-10-CM manual advises to use an additional code to identify which drug is causing the adverse effect. Identifying cyclosporine in the "Table of Drugs and Chemicals" leads to ICD-10-CM code T45.1X5, followed by the seventh character A to indicate active treatment. ICD-10CM code D63.9 (Anemia, unspecified) is listed as tertiary because this chronic underlying condition must be considered if the physician chooses to adjust the medication and/or treatment plan.

100. D: HACs are illnesses or injuries that arise from errors that could have been prevented by healthcare staff. Common HACs include infections due to bacteria exposure from a catheter, central line, or ventilator; postoperative fungal infections; hip fractures due to falls; pressure ulcers; and accidental lacerations during a surgical procedure. A foot ulcer arising from diabetes is not considered an HAC because it is usually the result of noncompliance to a medication or diet regime.

Medical Scenarios

Scenario #1

101. C, D, E, F, G: Foot pain, fatigue, muscle aches, and fevers are all symptoms of cellulitis, a skin infection. Neither of these codes should be reported because ICD-10-CM guidelines stipulate that when a definitive diagnosis is present, signs and/or symptoms should not be listed on the claim. Additionally, because skin infections, ulcers, and abscesses are common in patients who suffer from diabetes, E11.628 should be reported as a comorbidity. However, long-term/current use of oral hypoglycemic drugs should not be listed because the documentation does not specify how the diabetes is being managed.

102. B: Urgent care clinics follow the same rules regarding new versus established E/M procedure codes, even though the conditions are usually new. Beginning January 2021, outpatient E/M codes are leveled by time and/or the complexity of MDM, which includes the problems addressed, the data to be reviewed, and the risk of complications, morbidity, and/or mortality of patient management. In this scenario, the patient is suffering from an acute illness with systemic symptoms that include fatigue, muscle aches, and fevers. Additional treatment involves prescription drug management. Although the complexity of data reviewed is minimal, the other two elements suggest moderate MDM, making the most appropriate E/M code 99214.

Scenario #2

103. E: When sepsis is POA and meets the definition of principal diagnosis, it should be sequenced first, followed by the localized infection (e.g., pneumonia, urinary tract infection, etc.). However, if the sepsis originates from a procedure or the body's reaction to a prosthetic device, implant, or graft, a code from category T would be sequenced first, followed by the appropriate sepsis code. In an outpatient setting, diagnoses associated with the words "probable," "suspected," and "likely" should only be coded to their signs and/or symptoms; however, in an inpatient setting, these can be coded as if they were definitive.

104. C, D, F, G, H, I: The additional codes that should be reported are N39.0 (Urinary tract infection), B96.5 (Pseudomonas), I13.0 (Hypertensive heart and chronic kidney disease with heart failure and stage 1 through stage 4 chronic kidney disease, or unspecified chronic kidney disease), I50.23 (Acute on chronic systolic heart failure), and N18.2 (Chronic kidney disease stage II) and E78.5 (Hyperlipidemia). Chronic conditions and comorbidities should be reported as additional conditions because they must be monitored during an inpatient stay.

105. B: Because the patient was admitted into the hospital on the day prior to this encounter, a subsequent hospital E/M should be reported with CPT codes 99231–99233. When leveling this encounter, the following are some things to keep in mind:

- HPI: The history of present illness is quite limited, only stating the symptoms and when they began.
- EXAM: The documentation states that this was detailed.

- MDM: Sepsis is an acute illness that poses a threat to life because it can quickly lead to failure of several organ systems; however, the risk of morbidity is only moderate because the only diagnostic treatment taking place is prescription drug management.

All of these factors combined make the most appropriate reportable CPT code 99232.

Scenario #3

106. H: In the CPT manual index, locate "Anesthesia," followed by "Arthroplasty." An arthroplasty procedure was performed in order to correct a displaced condyle fracture related to the knee, thus arriving at CPT code 01402 (Anesthesia for open or surgical arthroscopic procedures on knee joint; total knee arthroplasty). Because 45 minutes were spent providing anesthesia services, three 15-minute time units should be reported, which may vary depending on the insurance carrier.

107. C, E, G: The correct codes that should be reported are S72.411A (Displaced unspecified condyle fracture of lower end of right femur, initial encounter for closed fracture), W19.XXXA (Accidental fall NOS), and Z99.3 (Dependence on wheelchair). A history of fractures should not be reported because further clarification is not provided on whether the fractures were traumatic or pathological. Additionally, any postprocedural state should not be reported because they are not indicative of the reason why the surgery took place.

Scenario #4

108. F: Critical care services can be rendered in any healthcare setting. Patients who are considered critical are defined by the CPT manual as "those with impairment to one or more vital organ systems with an increased risk of rapid or imminent health deterioration." In this scenario, because the patient has severe respiratory failure and kidney failure with an additional suspected systemic infection, all of which require high-complexity decision making in order to avoid further decline, CPT code 99291 (Critical care; first 30–74 minutes) may be reported. Because this code includes ventilation assistance, CPT 94660 (continuous positive airway pressure initiation and management) should not be reported as an additional service.

109. B: A principal diagnosis is not always the first-listed diagnosis in a medical chart; rather, it is the foremost reason for which the patient is receiving treatment in a hospital setting. Because the patient is being admitted for respiratory manifestations of the COVID-19 infection, the principal diagnosis code is U07.1 (COVID-19).

110. A, B, E, G: The correct additional codes that should be reported are J12.89 (Other viral pneumonia), J96.01 (Acute respiratory failure with hypoxia), N17.9 (Acute kidney failure), and N18.30 (Chronic kidney disease, stage 3 unspecified). Emergency rooms are considered outpatient settings; therefore, diseases that are listed as "probable" and "suspected" should only be coded to their signs and/or symptoms.

Scenario #5

111. E: As documented in the plan, the physician is admitting the patient into the hospital. Hospital admission codes are reported with CPT codes 99221-99223. However, when the documentation fails to meet the requirements of the lowest level in its category (which includes a detailed history, exam, and straightforward medical decision making), then CPT guidelines advise coders to use a subsequent inpatient care code (CPT codes 99231-99233).

To determine the level of service, review the documented history, examination, and medical decision making to find the following:

- HPI: The history of present illness is an expanded problem focus, only stating the timing of the symptoms and covering some review of systems.
- EXAM: The documentation supports a comprehensive examination.
- MDM: Diabetic ketoacidosis is an acute illness that poses a threat to life, as it produces a buildup of acids in the bloodstream that can force the body into a coma; however, the risk of morbidity is only moderate, as the only diagnostic treatment taking place is prescription drug management.

While the exam and medical decision making meet the documentation requirements of a hospital admission code, the documented history does not. Therefore, the two highest elements—the exam and medical decision making—can be used to select the appropriate subsequent inpatient care code (CPT code 99232).

112. A, D, E, F, G: The correct codes that should be reported are E11.10 (Type 2 diabetes mellitus with ketoacidosis without coma), E66.9 (Obesity, unspecified), I10 (Hypertension), Z79.4 (Long-term use of insulin), and Z68.42 (Body mass index 45.0–49.9, adult). Syncope, hypoglycemia, and abnormal blood glucose are all symptoms of diabetic ketoacidosis, which is due to a shortage of insulin in the body and should not be reported in lieu of a definitive diagnosis.

Scenario #6

113. B, E, F, G: The correct codes that should be reported are Z00.01 (Encounter for general adult medical examination with abnormal findings), Z23 (Encounter for immunization), E66.9 (Obesity, unspecified), and Z68.41 (Body mass index 40.0–44.9, adult). Although the patient's BMI is not documented in the assessment, it can be abstracted from the medical record when there is an associated and reportable diagnosis.

114. A, G, H: The correct codes that should be reported are 99396-25, 90471, and 90656. A preventative re-evaluation, otherwise known as an annual visit, is typically done to re-evaluate and manage the overall health condition of a patient. This may include recommendations based on personal risk factors, orders for laboratory and diagnostic testing, and an applicable history intake and examination. Although a separately identifiable E/M service may be appended to these services, time should not be the determining factor. CPT code G0008 should only be reported for Medicare patients receiving the flu vaccine.

Scenario #7

115. A: Although the underlying disease responsible for the admission is acute on chronic diastolic congestive heart failure (ICD-10-CM code I50.33), there is a "Code first" note for any causal conditions that may be associated with it. Because the patient has hypertension, and the documentation does not explicitly state that the two conditions are unrelated, hypertensive heart failure (ICD-10-CM code I11.0) should be the principal code.

116. A, B, D, G, H: The correct additional codes that should be reported are I25.10 (Coronary artery disease), Z86.73 (Personal history of stroke NOS without residual deficits), I50.33 (Acute on chronic diastolic congestive heart failure), E78.5 (Hyperlipidemia), and J96.01 (Acute respiratory failure with hypoxia). ICD-10-CM code I10 should not be coded alone because it has a causal relationship assumed with the heart failure.

117. F: The note describes hospital discharge management, which includes discharge instructions, a final patient evaluation, review of inpatient admission, final preparation of the patient's medical records, and provisional prescriptions/referrals. Hospital discharge management is reported with time spent with the patient, which, in this scenario, is greater than 30 minutes.

Scenario #8

118. A, H: The correct answer is 99283 and 16020. When billing for physician services in the emergency room, it is appropriate to report a stand-alone E/M when the documentation supports its necessity in determining the need for appropriate treatment. Modifier 25 is necessary to the E/M code when being billed alongside a procedure and/or surgery to indicate a separately billable service. In this case, the documentation supports an MDM of moderate complexity, which reflects CPT code 99283. The emergency room visit is always the first-listed code, followed by the procedure and/or surgery performed.

119. H: When the reason for admission is a burn, the site and severity of the burn (ICD-10-CM codes T20–T25) should be principal. The burns are considered to be second degree because they reached the dermis layer of the skin. The letter A is listed as the seventh character to T24.212, indicating that the injury and/or illness is actively being treated and is not yet in its recovery phase (a seventh character of D).

120. B, F, G, H: The correct answer is X08.8 (Exposure to other specified smoke), T31.0 (Burns involving less than 10% of the body), E11.9 (Type II diabetes), and Z79.84 (Long-term use of oral hypoglycemic drugs). When reporting diagnoses for burns, at least three codes are needed: the site and severity of the burn (ICD-10-CM codes T20–T25), the extent of the burn (ICD-10-CM codes T31–T32), and the external cause of the burn. Additionally, because the burns are caused by trauma, a causal relationship is not assumed between the two conditions and diabetes is coded as having no complications.

How to Overcome Test Anxiety

Just the thought of taking a test is enough to make most people a little nervous. A test is an important event that can have a long-term impact on your future, so it's important to take it seriously and it's natural to feel anxious about performing well. But just because anxiety is normal, that doesn't mean that it's helpful in test taking, or that you should simply accept it as part of your life. Anxiety can have a variety of effects. These effects can be mild, like making you feel slightly nervous, or severe, like blocking your ability to focus or remember even a simple detail.

If you experience test anxiety—whether severe or mild—it's important to know how to beat it. To discover this, first you need to understand what causes test anxiety.

Causes of Test Anxiety

While we often think of anxiety as an uncontrollable emotional state, it can actually be caused by simple, practical things. One of the most common causes of test anxiety is that a person does not feel adequately prepared for their test. This feeling can be the result of many different issues such as poor study habits or lack of organization, but the most common culprit is time management. Starting to study too late, failing to organize your study time to cover all of the material, or being distracted while you study will mean that you're not well prepared for the test. This may lead to cramming the night before, which will cause you to be physically and mentally exhausted for the test. Poor time management also contributes to feelings of stress, fear, and hopelessness as you realize you are not well prepared but don't know what to do about it.

Other times, test anxiety is not related to your preparation for the test but comes from unresolved fear. This may be a past failure on a test, or poor performance on tests in general. It may come from comparing yourself to others who seem to be performing better or from the stress of living up to expectations. Anxiety may be driven by fears of the future—how failure on this test would affect your educational and career goals. These fears are often completely irrational, but they can still negatively impact your test performance.

Review Video: 3 Reasons You Have Test Anxiety
Visit mometrix.com/academy and enter code: 428468

Elements of Test Anxiety

As mentioned earlier, test anxiety is considered to be an emotional state, but it has physical and mental components as well. Sometimes you may not even realize that you are suffering from test anxiety until you notice the physical symptoms. These can include trembling hands, rapid heartbeat, sweating, nausea, and tense muscles. Extreme anxiety may lead to fainting or vomiting. Obviously, any of these symptoms can have a negative impact on testing. It is important to recognize them as soon as they begin to occur so that you can address the problem before it damages your performance.

Review Video: 3 Ways to Tell You Have Test Anxiety
Visit mometrix.com/academy and enter code: 927847

The mental components of test anxiety include trouble focusing and inability to remember learned information. During a test, your mind is on high alert, which can help you recall information and stay focused for an extended period of time. However, anxiety interferes with your mind's natural processes, causing you to blank out, even on the questions you know well. The strain of testing during anxiety makes it difficult to stay focused, especially on a test that may take several hours. Extreme anxiety can take a huge mental toll, making it difficult not only to recall test information but even to understand the test questions or pull your thoughts together.

Review Video: How Test Anxiety Affects Memory
Visit mometrix.com/academy and enter code: 609003

Effects of Test Anxiety

Test anxiety is like a disease—if left untreated, it will get progressively worse. Anxiety leads to poor performance, and this reinforces the feelings of fear and failure, which in turn lead to poor performances on subsequent tests. It can grow from a mild nervousness to a crippling condition. If allowed to progress, test anxiety can have a big impact on your schooling, and consequently on your future.

Test anxiety can spread to other parts of your life. Anxiety on tests can become anxiety in any stressful situation, and blanking on a test can turn into panicking in a job situation. But fortunately, you don't have to let anxiety rule your testing and determine your grades. There are a number of relatively simple steps you can take to move past anxiety and function normally on a test and in the rest of life.

Review Video: How Test Anxiety Impacts Your Grades
Visit mometrix.com/academy and enter code: 939819

Physical Steps for Beating Test Anxiety

While test anxiety is a serious problem, the good news is that it can be overcome. It doesn't have to control your ability to think and remember information. While it may take time, you can begin taking steps today to beat anxiety.

Just as your first hint that you may be struggling with anxiety comes from the physical symptoms, the first step to treating it is also physical. Rest is crucial for having a clear, strong mind. If you are tired, it is much easier to give in to anxiety. But if you establish good sleep habits, your body and mind will be ready to perform optimally, without the strain of exhaustion. Additionally, sleeping well helps you to retain information better, so you're more likely to recall the answers when you see the test questions.

Getting good sleep means more than going to bed on time. It's important to allow your brain time to relax. Take study breaks from time to time so it doesn't get overworked, and don't study right before bed. Take time to rest your mind before trying to rest your body, or you may find it difficult to fall asleep.

Review Video: The Importance of Sleep for Your Brain
Visit mometrix.com/academy and enter code: 319338

Along with sleep, other aspects of physical health are important in preparing for a test. Good nutrition is vital for good brain function. Sugary foods and drinks may give a burst of energy but this burst is followed by a crash, both physically and emotionally. Instead, fuel your body with protein and vitamin-rich foods.

Also, drink plenty of water. Dehydration can lead to headaches and exhaustion, especially if your brain is already under stress from the rigors of the test. Particularly if your test is a long one, drink water during the breaks. And if possible, take an energy-boosting snack to eat between sections.

Review Video: How Diet Can Affect your Mood
Visit mometrix.com/academy and enter code: 624317

Along with sleep and diet, a third important part of physical health is exercise. Maintaining a steady workout schedule is helpful, but even taking 5-minute study breaks to walk can help get your blood pumping faster and clear your head. Exercise also releases endorphins, which contribute to a positive feeling and can help combat test anxiety.

When you nurture your physical health, you are also contributing to your mental health. If your body is healthy, your mind is much more likely to be healthy as well. So take time to rest, nourish your body with healthy food and water, and get moving as much as possible. Taking these physical steps will make you stronger and more able to take the mental steps necessary to overcome test anxiety.

Mental Steps for Beating Test Anxiety

Working on the mental side of test anxiety can be more challenging, but as with the physical side, there are clear steps you can take to overcome it. As mentioned earlier, test anxiety often stems from lack of preparation, so the obvious solution is to prepare for the test. Effective studying may be the most important weapon you have for beating test anxiety, but you can and should employ several other mental tools to combat fear.

First, boost your confidence by reminding yourself of past success—tests or projects that you aced. If you're putting as much effort into preparing for this test as you did for those, there's no reason you should expect to fail here. Work hard to prepare; then trust your preparation.

Second, surround yourself with encouraging people. It can be helpful to find a study group, but be sure that the people you're around will encourage a positive attitude. If you spend time with others who are anxious or cynical, this will only contribute to your own anxiety. Look for others who are motivated to study hard from a desire to succeed, not from a fear of failure.

Third, reward yourself. A test is physically and mentally tiring, even without anxiety, and it can be helpful to have something to look forward to. Plan an activity following the test, regardless of the outcome, such as going to a movie or getting ice cream.

When you are taking the test, if you find yourself beginning to feel anxious, remind yourself that you know the material. Visualize successfully completing the test. Then take a few deep, relaxing breaths and return to it. Work through the questions carefully but with confidence, knowing that you are capable of succeeding.

Developing a healthy mental approach to test taking will also aid in other areas of life. Test anxiety affects more than just the actual test—it can be damaging to your mental health and even contribute to depression. It's important to beat test anxiety before it becomes a problem for more than testing.

Review Video: Test Anxiety and Depression
Visit mometrix.com/academy and enter code: 904704

Study Strategy

Being prepared for the test is necessary to combat anxiety, but what does being prepared look like? You may study for hours on end and still not feel prepared. What you need is a strategy for test prep. The next few pages outline our recommended steps to help you plan out and conquer the challenge of preparation.

Step 1: Scope Out the Test

Learn everything you can about the format (multiple choice, essay, etc.) and what will be on the test. Gather any study materials, course outlines, or sample exams that may be available. Not only will this help you to prepare, but knowing what to expect can help to alleviate test anxiety.

Step 2: Map Out the Material

Look through the textbook or study guide and make note of how many chapters or sections it has. Then divide these over the time you have. For example, if a book has 15 chapters and you have five days to study, you need to cover three chapters each day. Even better, if you have the time, leave an extra day at the end for overall review after you have gone through the material in depth.

If time is limited, you may need to prioritize the material. Look through it and make note of which sections you think you already have a good grasp on, and which need review. While you are studying, skim quickly through the familiar sections and take more time on the challenging parts. Write out your plan so you don't get lost as you go. Having a written plan also helps you feel more in control of the study, so anxiety is less likely to arise from feeling overwhelmed at the amount to cover.

Step 3: Gather Your Tools

Decide what study method works best for you. Do you prefer to highlight in the book as you study and then go back over the highlighted portions? Or do you type out notes of the important information? Or is it helpful to make flashcards that you can carry with you? Assemble the pens, index cards, highlighters, post-it notes, and any other materials you may need so you won't be distracted by getting up to find things while you study.

If you're having a hard time retaining the information or organizing your notes, experiment with different methods. For example, try color-coding by subject with colored pens, highlighters, or post-it notes. If you learn better by hearing, try recording yourself reading your notes so you can listen while in the car, working out, or simply sitting at your desk. Ask a friend to quiz you from your flashcards, or try teaching someone the material to solidify it in your mind.

Step 4: Create Your Environment

It's important to avoid distractions while you study. This includes both the obvious distractions like visitors and the subtle distractions like an uncomfortable chair (or a too-comfortable couch that makes you want to fall asleep). Set up the best study environment possible: good lighting and a comfortable work area. If background music helps you focus, you may want to turn it on, but otherwise keep the room quiet. If you are using a computer to take notes, be sure you don't have any other windows open, especially applications like social media, games, or anything else that could distract you. Silence your phone and turn off notifications. Be sure to keep water close by so you stay hydrated while you study (but avoid unhealthy drinks and snacks).

Also, take into account the best time of day to study. Are you freshest first thing in the morning? Try to set aside some time then to work through the material. Is your mind clearer in the afternoon or evening? Schedule your study session then. Another method is to study at the same time of day that you will take the test, so that your brain gets used to working on the material at that time and will be ready to focus at test time.

Step 5: Study!

Once you have done all the study preparation, it's time to settle into the actual studying. Sit down, take a few moments to settle your mind so you can focus, and begin to follow your study plan. Don't give in to distractions or let yourself procrastinate. This is your time to prepare so you'll be ready to fearlessly approach the test. Make the most of the time and stay focused.

Of course, you don't want to burn out. If you study too long you may find that you're not retaining the information very well. Take regular study breaks. For example, taking five minutes out of every hour to walk briskly, breathing deeply and swinging your arms, can help your mind stay fresh.

As you get to the end of each chapter or section, it's a good idea to do a quick review. Remind yourself of what you learned and work on any difficult parts. When you feel that you've mastered the material, move on to the next part. At the end of your study session, briefly skim through your notes again.

But while review is helpful, cramming last minute is NOT. If at all possible, work ahead so that you won't need to fit all your study into the last day. Cramming overloads your brain with more information than it can process and retain, and your tired mind may struggle to recall even previously learned information when it is overwhelmed with last-minute study. Also, the urgent nature of cramming and the stress placed on your brain contribute to anxiety. You'll be more likely to go to the test feeling unprepared and having trouble thinking clearly.

So don't cram, and don't stay up late before the test, even just to review your notes at a leisurely pace. Your brain needs rest more than it needs to go over the information again. In fact, plan to finish your studies by noon or early afternoon the day before the test. Give your brain the rest of the day to relax or focus on other things, and get a good night's sleep. Then you will be fresh for the test and better able to recall what you've studied.

Step 6: Take a Practice Test

Many courses offer sample tests, either online or in the study materials. This is an excellent resource to check whether you have mastered the material, as well as to prepare for the test format and environment.

Check the test format ahead of time: the number of questions, the type (multiple choice, free response, etc.), and the time limit. Then create a plan for working through them. For example, if you have 30 minutes to take a 60-question test, your limit is 30 seconds per question. Spend less time on the questions you know well so that you can take more time on the difficult ones.

If you have time to take several practice tests, take the first one open book, with no time limit. Work through the questions at your own pace and make sure you fully understand them. Gradually work up to taking a test under test conditions: sit at a desk with all study materials put away and set a timer. Pace yourself to make sure you finish the test with time to spare and go back to check your answers if you have time.

After each test, check your answers. On the questions you missed, be sure you understand why you missed them. Did you misread the question (tests can use tricky wording)? Did you forget the information? Or was it something you hadn't learned? Go back and study any shaky areas that the practice tests reveal.

Taking these tests not only helps with your grade, but also aids in combating test anxiety. If you're already used to the test conditions, you're less likely to worry about it, and working through tests until you're scoring well gives you a confidence boost. Go through the practice tests until you feel comfortable, and then you can go into the test knowing that you're ready for it.

Test Tips

On test day, you should be confident, knowing that you've prepared well and are ready to answer the questions. But aside from preparation, there are several test day strategies you can employ to maximize your performance.

First, as stated before, get a good night's sleep the night before the test (and for several nights before that, if possible). Go into the test with a fresh, alert mind rather than staying up late to study.

Try not to change too much about your normal routine on the day of the test. It's important to eat a nutritious breakfast, but if you normally don't eat breakfast at all, consider eating just a protein bar. If you're a coffee drinker, go ahead and have your normal coffee. Just make sure you time it so that the caffeine doesn't wear off right in the middle of your test. Avoid sugary beverages, and drink enough water to stay hydrated but not so much that you need a restroom break 10 minutes into the test. If your test isn't first thing in the morning, consider going for a walk or doing a light workout before the test to get your blood flowing.

Allow yourself enough time to get ready, and leave for the test with plenty of time to spare so you won't have the anxiety of scrambling to arrive in time. Another reason to be early is to select a good seat. It's helpful to sit away from doors and windows, which can be distracting. Find a good seat, get out your supplies, and settle your mind before the test begins.

When the test begins, start by going over the instructions carefully, even if you already know what to expect. Make sure you avoid any careless mistakes by following the directions.

Then begin working through the questions, pacing yourself as you've practiced. If you're not sure on an answer, don't spend too much time on it, and don't let it shake your confidence. Either skip it and come back later, or eliminate as many wrong answers as possible and guess among the remaining ones. Don't dwell on these questions as you continue—put them out of your mind and focus on what lies ahead.

Be sure to read all of the answer choices, even if you're sure the first one is the right answer. Sometimes you'll find a better one if you keep reading. But don't second-guess yourself if you do immediately know the answer. Your gut instinct is usually right. Don't let test anxiety rob you of the information you know.

If you have time at the end of the test (and if the test format allows), go back and review your answers. Be cautious about changing any, since your first instinct tends to be correct, but make sure you didn't misread any of the questions or accidentally mark the wrong answer choice. Look over any you skipped and make an educated guess.

At the end, leave the test feeling confident. You've done your best, so don't waste time worrying about your performance or wishing you could change anything. Instead, celebrate the successful completion of this test. And finally, use this test to learn how to deal with anxiety even better next time.

Review Video: 5 Tips to Beat Test Anxiety
Visit mometrix.com/academy and enter code: 570656

Important Qualification

Not all anxiety is created equal. If your test anxiety is causing major issues in your life beyond the classroom or testing center, or if you are experiencing troubling physical symptoms related to your anxiety, it may be a sign of a serious physiological or psychological condition. If this sounds like your situation, we strongly encourage you to seek professional help.

Thank You

We at Mometrix would like to extend our heartfelt thanks to you, our friend and patron, for allowing us to play a part in your journey. It is a privilege to serve people from all walks of life who are unified in their commitment to building the best future they can for themselves.

The preparation you devote to these important testing milestones may be the most valuable educational opportunity you have for making a real difference in your life. We encourage you to put your heart into it—that feeling of succeeding, overcoming, and yes, conquering will be well worth the hours you've invested.

We want to hear your story, your struggles and your successes, and if you see any opportunities for us to improve our materials so we can help others even more effectively in the future, please share that with us as well. **The team at Mometrix would be absolutely thrilled to hear from you!** So please, send us an email (support@mometrix.com) and let's stay in touch.

If you'd like some additional help, check out these other resources we offer for your exam: http://mometrixflashcards.com/AHIMA

Additional Bonus Material

Due to our efforts to try to keep this book to a manageable length, we've created a link that will give you access to all of your additional bonus material.

Please visit https://www.mometrix.com/bonus948/certcodespec to access the information.